T0360427

Economics of Tobacco Control in China

From Policy Research to Practice

World Scientific Series in Global Health Economics and Public Policy

ISSN: 2010-2089

Series Editor-in-Chief: Richard M Scheffler
University of California, Berkeley, USA

Published:

Vol. 1   Accountability and Responsibility in Health Care:
Issues in Addressing an Emerging Global Challenge
edited by Bruce Rosen, Avi Israeli and Stephen Shortell

Vol. 2   The Economics of Social Capital and Health:
A Conceptual and Empirical Roadmap
edited by Sherman Folland and Lorenzo Rocco

Vol. 3   World Scientific Handbook of Global Health Economics and Public Policy
edited by Richard M Scheffler

Vol. 4   Economics of Tobacco Control in China: From Policy Research to Practice
edited by Teh-wei Hu

World Scientific Series in Global Healthcare Economics and Public Policy — Vol. 4

Economics of Tobacco Control in China

From Policy Research to Practice

Edited by

Teh-wei Hu

University of California, Berkeley, USA

World Scientific

NEW JERSEY · LONDON · SINGAPORE · BEIJING · SHANGHAI · HONG KONG · TAIPEI · CHENNAI · TOKYO

Published by

World Scientific Publishing Co. Pte. Ltd.
5 Toh Tuck Link, Singapore 596224
USA office: 27 Warren Street, Suite 401-402, Hackensack, NJ 07601
UK office: 57 Shelton Street, Covent Garden, London WC2H 9HE

Library of Congress Cataloging-in-Publication Data
Names: Hu, Teh-wei, editor.
Title: Economics of tobacco control in China : from policy research to practice /
    [edited by] Teh-wei Hu.
Other titles: World Scientific series in global healthcare economics and
    public policy ; v. 4. 2010-2089
Description: New Jersey : World Scientific, 2016. | Series: World Scientific
    series in global health economics and public policy ; vol. 4 |
    Includes bibliographical references and index.
Identifiers: LCCN 2016009431 | ISBN 9789813108714 (hardcover : alk. paper)
Subjects: | MESH: Tobacco Use Disorder--prevention & control |
    Tobacco Use Disorder--economics | Health Policy | Tobacco Use Cessation--economics |
    Tobacco Products--economics | China
Classification: LCC RA1242.T6 | NLM WM 290 | DDC 362.19686/500951--dc23
LC record available at http://lccn.loc.gov/2016009431

British Library Cataloguing-in-Publication Data
A catalogue record for this book is available from the British Library.

Desk Editor: Qi Xiao

Typeset by Stallion Press
Email: enquiries@stallionpress.com

Printed in Singapore

Preface

At the 2004 World Health Organization (WHO) Framework Convention on Tobacco Control meeting, former Director General of the WHO, Gro Harlem Brundtland, stated: "Health, not economic arguments, are the reasons for controlling tobacco, but economic arguments are raised as an obstacle to tobacco control policies." Indeed it is very important for tobacco control professionals and government policymakers to understand the economic issues of tobacco control in order to face challenges from the tobacco industry. About eight years ago, I edited a book titled *Tobacco Control Policy Analysis in China: Economics and Health*, published by World Scientific Publishing (2007). That book addressed why the Chinese government should raise the tobacco tax and analyzed the demand for and the supply of tobacco in China.

This book is a continuation of the first book. It addresses not only why China should raise the cigarette tax, but also *how* to raise the tobacco tax. It provides quantitative estimates to show that raising the tobacco tax is indeed a win-win public policy that the increased tax can reduce the smoking prevalence rate, saving lives and medical care costs, improve society's economic productivity, and also raise government revenue. By providing decision makers with relevant research findings and quantitative estimates about the impact of raising the tobacco tax, tobacco tax reform can more easily be implemented.

After conducting research on the economics of tobacco control for almost 25 years (since the early 1990s), it was rather rewarding to witness the Chinese government finally raising taxes on cigarette products in May 2015. Most gratifying was that, unlike the tax increase in 2009 which raised prices at the producer and wholesale levels, this latest tax increase was passed on to the retail price level. One unique feature of this book is to document how our research team disseminated our policy findings to Chinese government officials from mid-level government officials responsible for policy design and policy implementation to the highest government leaders who initiate the policy decisions. The book also addresses how media can be very helpful in influencing decision makers. This Chinese case study could be useful for tobacco control professionals and public policy researchers in other countries.

During the past 15 years, many organizations have supported the work reported in this book. These include the Bloomberg Philanthropies, the Gates Foundation, and particularly the National Institutes of Health, Fogarty International Center and National Cancer Institute (RO1-TW009295). We are very grateful for three consecutive five-year (2002–2017) funding grants from NIH to conduct this research on the economics of tobacco control in China. We are now in the fourteenth year. Therefore, this book can be considered as a fruit of this NIH funding.

In addition to funding institutions, I am most grateful to many of my colleagues who contributed to this book, especially Professor Zhengzhong Mao at Sichuan University, with whom I have collaborated for more than 25 years, Dr. Anita Lee who has been my valuable colleague at the Public Health Institute during the past 8 years, and Professor Xiulan Zhang at the Beijing Normal University who during the past 2 years mobilized her network in the Chinese government to promote our research findings. Thanks to D. Lynne Kaltreider, formerly with The Pennsylvania State University, who provided excellent editing not only of this book, but also of my writings throughout my 45-year professional career. Thanks to Dr. Xingzhu Liu, formerly at the Fogarty International Center, for his encouragement and support for our tobacco research projects. I wish to acknowledge my two assistants, Michelle Lan and Vivian Wu at the University of California, Berkeley, for organizing this volume so well. I am grateful to Ms. Hongyan Li and Mr. Xiao Qi for their production services at the World Scientific Publishing Company. Finally I thank my wife Tien-hwa for her patient support and understanding, as I was away from home many days for this project during these past 25 years. I am forever grateful.

Teh-wei Hu
Berkeley, California
December 2015

Contents

List of Contributors

Teh-wei Hu
School of Public Health
University of California
Berkeley, CA, USA
and
Public Health Institute
Oakland, CA, USA

Elizabeth D. Brouwer
Department of Global Health
University of Washington
Seattle, WA, USA

Wendong Chen
Research Institute of Taxation Science
State Administration of Taxation
Beijing, China

Yuyu Chen
Guanghua School of management
Beijing University
Beijing, China

Geoffrey T. Fong
Department of Psychology
University of Waterloo
Ontario, Canada

Song Gao
School of Taxation
Central University of Finance and Taxation
Beijing, China

Cindy L. Gauvreau
Department of Global Health
University of Washington
Seattle, WA, USA

Dean T. Jamison
Global Health Sciences
University of California
San Francisco, CA, USA

Pradhat Jha
Center for Global Health Research
University of Toronto
Toronto, Ontario, Canada

Yuan Jiang
Tobacco Control Office
China Center for Disease Control and Prevention
Beijing, China

Anita H. Lee
Public Health Institute
Oakland, CA, USA

David Levy
Department of Oncology
Georgetown University
Washington DC, USA

Jing Li
School of Public Health
University of California
Berkeley, CA, USA

Steve Lin
School of Social Development and Public Policy
Beijing Normal University
Beijing, China

Mary MacLennan
Center for Global Health Research
University of Toronto
Toronto, Ontario, Canada

Zhengzhong Mao
Department of Health Economics
Sichuan University
Chengdu, Sichuan, China

Wendy Max
Institute for Health and Aging
University of California
San Francisco, CA, USA

Sujata Mishra
Center for Global Health Research
University of Toronto
Toronto, Ontario, Canada

Andrew E. Moran
Columbia University Medical Center
Columbia University, New York, USA

Rachel A. Nugent
Department of Global Health
University of Washington
Seattle, WA, USA

Keqin Rao
Center for Health Statistics of Information
Chinese Ministry of Health
Beijing, China

Ricardo L. Rodriquez-Buno
University de Granada
Granada, Spain

Jian Shi
Research Institute of Taxation Science
State Administration of Taxation
Beijing, China

Hai-yen Sung
Institute for Health and Aging
University of California
San Francisco, CA, USA

Stephane Verguet
Department of Global Health and Population
Harvard University
Boston, MA, USA

Justin S. White
School of Medicine
University of California
San Francisco, CA, USA

Weibo Xing
Department of Public Finance and Taxation
University of International Business and Economics
Beijing, China

Lian Yang
School of Public Health and Administration
Chengdu University of Traditional Chinese Medicine
Chengdu, Sichuan, China

Tingting Yao
Institute for Health and Aging
University of California
San Francisco, CA, USA

Xiulan Zhang
School of Social Development and Public Policy
Beijing Normal University
Beijing, China

Kun Zhao
National Health Development Research Center
Beijing, China

Rong Zheng
WHO Coordinating Center for Tobacco Control
University of International Business and Economics
Beijing, China

Introduction

Teh-wei Hu

China has a population of more than 1.3 billion. Nearly 370 million people in China smoke; about one-third of all smokers in the world are in China. About 65 percent of those who do not smoke, mostly women and children, are exposed to harmful second-hand smoke (SHS). The negative health consequences of smoking include more than 1.2 million smoking-related deaths in China each year. If smoking rates in China do not decrease, the smoking death toll in China by the year 2030 is expected to be more than 2.2 million people per year. Cigarette smoking is a driving force in the rising rate of chronic diseases in China, a situation that puts increasing pressure on China's economy and its health care system.

One of the major challenges of tobacco control in China is the Chinese tobacco industry. The Chinese tobacco industry is a government-owned national monopoly, the China State Tobacco Monopoly Administration (STMA). STMA is the world's largest tobacco producer controlling more than 40% of the global market. In 2014, STMA contributed close to US$130 billion as tax to the Chinese central government, about 6.7% of total government tax revenue. The importance of STMA in the Chinese economy has caused strong opposing views about tobacco control within the Chinese government. Therefore, tobacco control in China is both a health issue and an economic issue. This book addresses the economic aspects of tobacco control in China.

The articles included in this book show that using taxes as a tobacco control policy is a win-win policy instrument. Increased taxes will not only generate more government revenue, but will also help to reduce the smoking prevalence rate, which will lead to better health for China's population.

The purposes of this book are (1) to inform economists, public health professionals, and policymakers about the economic consequences of smoking, (2) to provide the essential economics (particularly related to taxation) and public health information upon which to build the specifics of the taxation policy that is adopted, (3) to identify barriers, challenges, and recommendations for the Chinese government, and (4) to describe how research findings can be disseminated and communicated successfully to Chinese government policy makers. The book constitutes a rather rare case study that, since 1990, the authors continuously participated in tobacco control policy research and sent in annual policy recommendations to the Chinese government officials. Finally, after 25 years, Chinese government adopted some of their recommendations in 2015.

The book is divided into four sections. Section I provides estimates of the economic costs of smoking in China, incurred by both smokers and secondhand smokers. Section II analyzes the demand for cigarettes, including smokers' brand switches in response to price changes. Section III describes the Chinese tobacco taxation system and analyzes the impact of tax adjustments on the Chinese economy and population health. Section IV, the final section, presents barriers and challenges to tobacco control and describes how research findings have been disseminated to government officials and media with recommendations for implementing tobacco control policy in China. The book contains 14 chapters in addition to this introductory chapter.

Section I has three chapters. One of the economic consequences of smoking is the increased health care costs and the cost of premature deaths attributable to smoking. Chapter 2 estimates the direct health care costs attributable to smoking as US$6.2 billion in 2008, accounting for 3.0% of total national health care costs in China. The 2008 costs represent an increase of 154% over the US$2.4 billion costs in the year 2000. The indirect mortality cost associated with smoking in China was US$22.0 billion in 2008, an increase of 376% over 2000 costs (US$4.2 billion). These economic costs of smoking have increased substantially during the past decade. Stronger intervention measures against smoking should be implemented without delay.

Chapter 3 estimates that based on data from the 2008 China National Rural Household Survey, secondhand smoke exposure at home in rural China was 68% for children and about 60% for women. The exposure was more serious for lower socioeconomic households. The great need to reduce this exposure could be met by designing tobacco control intervention programs. Chapter 4 uses data from the 2011 Chinese National Rural Household Survey of adults in rural China to estimate the health care cost of secondhand smoking in rural China. The total health care cost of SHS exposure in rural China was about US$1.20 billion in 2011, including US$559 million for outpatient visits and US$612 million for inpatient hospitalization. The total health care cost of SHS exposure in rural China accounted for 0.3% of China's national health care costs in 2011.

Section II contains four chapters. Chapter 5 estimates the price elasticity of cigarettes, using data for 1999–2001 from an urban household survey in China. The estimated price elasticities range from −0.35 to −0.81, depending on the price and quality of cigarettes. These estimated price elasticities suggest that if the tobacco excise tax rate goes up, cigarette consumption will drop rapidly, and government revenue from the tobacco tax will increase.

Chapters 6 and 7 both address the issue of the effectiveness of the tobacco tax on demand for cigarettes in China. China has a wide price range of cigarettes, from US$0.20 to $10.00 per pack. Chinese government leaders claim that smokers may simply switch to cheaper brands when the price of cigarettes increases due to a tax increase. Thus, they argue, raising the cigarette tax may not be that effective in tobacco control. Two studies used longitudinal data from the International Tobacco Control China Survey collected in six large Chinese cities between 2006 and 2009 to estimate how cigarette price changes would influence smokers' choice of cigarette brands in China. Chapter 6 reports that a 1 RMB (US$0.15) change in the price of cigarettes altered the choice of brands by one tier (brands in China are classified into five tiers, from high to low prices) of 4–7% of smokers. That is, tobacco pricing and tax policy can influence smokers' incentives to switch to a cheaper (lower-tier) brand, but to a limited amount. However, it should be noted that ad valorem taxes, the percentage tax rates of which are based on product price, are more likely to encourage smokers to trade down, while specific excise taxes, a fixed amount of tax based on product quantity, discourage the practice. Chapter 7 uses the same data set to examine how different socioeconomic subgroups of

Chinese smokers switch brands in response to cigarette price changes. The analysis found that low-income smokers were more likely to switch brands than their high-income counterparts — about 5.6% of low-income smokers compared to 1.6% of high-income smokers. However, no matter how the groups were classified, the magnitude of brand switching was relatively low. Hence, the concern of the Chinese government officials that a tax increase will lead to a large-scale brand switch was not supported by these two studies.

One of the challenges China faces in implementing tobacco control policies is to change the social norm, especially the culture and behaviors surrounding cigarette gift giving. Chapter 8 uses data from the 2005 National Tobacco Use Survey collected by the China National Bureau of Statistics, which surveyed 50,000 rural and urban households. The analysis found that government workers, teachers, and physicians constituted the largest group (32% respectively) to receive cigarettes as gifts. Business owners, young adults (ages 15–19), teachers, physicians, and military personnel comprised the largest group (between 10–13%) to give cigarettes as gifts. Tobacco control measures should be aimed at changing the cigarette gifting culture and behavior in China. In November 2013, the Chinese government released a regulation that prohibited giving cigarettes as gifts to government officials, a major step toward changing the social norm away from using cigarettes as a means of gift giving.

Section III includes five chapters on the Chinese tobacco taxation system and the impact of reform. Chapter 9 first describes the tobacco economy in China, the tobacco tax system and tax structure in China, and then uses the estimated price elasticities of the demand for cigarettes to simulate the potential impact of the increased tobacco tax on government revenue and population health, and the impact on employment in the cigarette industry and tobacco farming. At a price elasticity of −0.15, a tax increase of 1 RMB (US$0.13) per pack of cigarettes would increase Chinese government revenue by 129 billion RMB (US$17.2 billion), decrease consumption by 3.0 billion packs of cigarettes, reduce the number of smokers by 3.42 million, and save 1.14 million lives. This finding has been extensively quoted by the international tobacco control organizations (WHO, World Bank, and the International Union against Tuberculosis and Lung Diseases), and by media as a strong justification for the Chinese government to raise the tobacco tax.

In 2009 China raised the ad valorem tax at the producer price level and the tax at the wholesale price level, but it did not transfer these increased taxes to retail prices. Chapter 10 compares the pre- and post-2009 new tobacco tax structure and simulates the potential impact on tobacco control if the new tobacco tax structure were transferred to the retail prices. Once again this paper recommends that the Chinese government raise the specific excise tax and eliminate the two-tier ad valorem tax, replacing it with a uniform tax rate.

Chapter 11 is a follow-up essay to explain China's cigarette pricing mechanism and the role of the China State Monopoly Administration (STMA) in cigarette pricing and taxation. China's tobacco industry is not a market economy; therefore, nonmarket forces and the current Chinese tobacco monopoly system determine cigarette retail prices. Because the STMA did not want to reduce its national cigarette sales volume, the 2009 tax increase did not get passed on from the producer and wholesale level to the retail prices.

Chapter 12 is an extension of Chapter 9, and uses a Markov computer simulation model (SimSmoke) to predict the impact of implementing the key interventions of the WHO Framework Convention on Tobacco Control (FCTC): tobacco tax, smoke-free law, strong warning label, ban of cigarette advertisements, and cessation treatment. The study used 1991–2010 tobacco smoking prevalence data in China to predict the long-term impact of these key interventions. The results showed that complete implementation of all these WHO-FCTC recommended policies would prevent more than 12.8 million smoking attributable deaths, or 154 million life years in China by 2050. Among these individual recommended tobacco control measures, raising the tobacco tax up to 75% of the retail price is one of the most effective policy measures. This one measure would save 3.48 million lives and would account for about 27% of the total effects of tobacco control policy.

Chapter 13 uses cost-effectiveness analysis to estimate the impact of raising tobacco prices by 50% through an excise tax. About 231 million years of life would be gained over 50 years, one-third of which could be gained in the lowest income quintiles. The government would also receive US$703 billion in additional revenue from this excise tax increase. This chapter concludes that increased tobacco taxation can be a "pro-poor" policy instrument that brings substantial health and financial benefits to households in China.

Section IV contains two chapters. Chapter 14 was prepared three years after the Chinese government introduced the 2009 tobacco tax adjustment which did not shift the increased tax to cigarette retail prices. The authors examine the barriers and challenges of moving tobacco control policies forward under the Chinese government. This chapter recommends both top-down and bottom-up approaches under the current Chinese political system to mobilize tobacco control forces.

Chapter 15 documents the processes used to disseminate the policy research findings to Chinese government middle-level as well as top political leaders. It also describes how this information was shared with Chinese media networks. This chapter includes a policy brief that was submitted to the President's office. A final section of this chapter illustrates the successful result of linking policy research to policy adoption with further policy recommendations for the next stage of tobacco control and tobacco tax increases in China.

Section I
Economic Costs of Smoking

Chapter 2

Economic Costs Attributable to Smoking in China: Update and an 8-year Comparison, 2000–2008*

Lian Yang, Hai-Yen Sung, Zhengzhong Mao,
Teh-wei Hu and Keqin Rao

ABSTRACT

Objective — To estimate the health-related economic costs attributable to smoking in China for persons aged 35 and older in 2003 and in 2008 and to compare these costs with the respective results from 2000.

Methods — A prevalence-based, disease-specific approach was used to estimate smoking-attributable direct and indirect economic costs. The primary data source was the 2003 and 2008 China National Health Services Survey, which contains individual participant's smoking status, healthcare utilization, and expenditures.

Results — The total economic cost of smoking in China amounted to $17.1 billion in 2003 and $28.9 billion in 2008 (both measured in 2008 constant US dollars). Direct smoking-attributable healthcare costs in 2003 and 2008 were $4.2 billion and $6.2 billion, respectively. Indirect economic costs in 2003 and 2008 were $12.9 billion and $22.7 billion, respectively. Compared to 2000, the direct costs of smoking

*Published in *Tob Control*, 2011; 20(4): 266–272. doi: 10.1136/tc.2010.042028 (July, 2011).

rose by 72% in 2003 and 154% in 2008, while the indirect costs of smoking rose by 170% in 2003 and 376% in 2008.

Conclusion — The economic burden of cigarette smoking has increased substantially in China during the past decade and is expected to continue to increase as the national economy and the price of healthcare services grow. Stronger intervention measures against smoking should be taken without delay to reduce the health and financial losses caused by smoking.

INTRODUCTION

With 301 million current smokers in 2010, [1] China is the largest consumer of tobacco in the world. In 2010, 52.9% of Chinese men and 2.4% of women were current smokers. Despite numerous studies demonstrating that tobacco is harmful for health [2–5] and evidence showing that the overall mortality of smokers in China is significantly higher than that of never smokers, [6] most Chinese still lack understanding of the harmful effects of smoking. In 2010, only 23.2% of Chinese adults believed smoking causes stroke, heart attack, and lung cancer, and only 16.1% of current smokers planned to or were thinking about quitting in the next 12 months [1].

At the same time, China is the world's largest producer of tobacco. All cigarettes are produced by the state-owned tobacco monopoly company, and about 7.0% of China's central government revenue was generated from tobacco profit and taxes [7]. Because of the economic interests of the tobacco industry, Chinese policymakers are unwilling to restrict promotion of tobacco products and to implement stricter legislation to protect non-smokers. To raise the general Chinese population's awareness of the dangers of smoking and to increase the government's incentive to implement the promises of the ratified World Health Organization's Framework Convention on Tobacco Control, it is important to transform the data on the health effects of smoking into monetary values of financial losses to the society.

There is a paucity of national studies estimating the economic costs of smoking in China. Using a medical cost accounting method to calculate disease-specific medical costs, Chen *et al.* [8] estimated the total medical costs attributable to smoking in 1988 in China at 2.3 billion Yuan (US$0.28 billion using the exchange rate of 8.2784 Yuan to US$1). Jin *et al.* [9] estimated the total economic burden of smoking in China in 1989 at 27.1 billion Yuan ($3.27 billion using the exchange rate of 8.2784 Yuan to US$1), including

6.9 billion Yuan ($0.83 billion) of direct medical costs and 20.1 billion Yuan ($2.43 billion) of indirect morbidity and mortality costs. Sung *et al.* [10] estimated the economic costs of smoking in China in 2000 at $5.0 billion (based on the exchange rate of 8.2784 Yuan to US$1), of which $1.7 billion were direct healthcare costs of smoking and $3.3 billion were indirect morbidity and mortality costs. These three studies of the costs of smoking in China were conducted more than ten years ago. Due to China's economic growth and the introduction of high-tech medical equipment, wage rates and healthcare expenditures in China have increased substantially during the last decade. Therefore, the economic burden of smoking in China is very likely to have increased dramatically as well. It is important to examine the trend of smoking-attributable costs during the last decade.

The objective of this paper is to provide the latest estimates for both direct and indirect costs of smoking in China by using data from the third and fourth waves of the China National Health Services Survey (NHSS) conducted in 2003 and 2008 and to compare these cost estimates with the respective 2000 estimates from the previous study by Sung *et al.* [10].

METHODS

We divided the economic costs of smoking into two components: direct costs and indirect costs. Direct costs include all healthcare expenditures for treating smoking-related diseases. Indirect costs include expenses for transportation, nutritious supplemental food, and caregivers during inpatient hospitalizations and outpatient visits due to treating smoking-related diseases, the value of lost productivity caused by smoking-related illness, and indirect mortality costs of premature deaths caused by smoking-related diseases. Healthcare services comprise outpatient visits, inpatient hospitalizations, and self-medication. We used the prevalence-based, disease-specific approach to measure the costs of smoking-related diseases and deaths in a given year (2003 or 2008) caused by current and past smoking. Three kinds of smoking-related diseases were included: cancer (ICD–10:C00–C97), cardiovascular diseases (ICD–10:I00–I99), and respiratory diseases (ICD–10:J00–J99). Because the average age at uptake for Chinese smokers was 21 years old, [11] and because smoking-related diseases usually occur after having smoked for a long time, we included only adults aged 35+ in the analysis [12].

Smoking-attributable Fraction (SAF)

We calculated the SAF for each component of the economic burden of smoking by disease category, rural/urban district, gender, and age. Levin [13, 14] developed the formula for "attributable risk" to examine the proportion of lung cancer cases attributable to cigarette smoking. Attributable risk was first renamed the smoking-attributable fraction (SAF) in a computer software program, Smoking-Attributable Mortality, Morbidity, and Economic Cost (SAMMEC) [15–17]. The SAF is specified by the following epidemiological formula:

$$SAF_{irsa} \frac{(PN_{rsa} + PS_{rsa} \times RR_{irsa}) - 1}{(PN_{rsa} + PS_{rsa} + RR_{irsa})} \tag{1}$$

where PN and PS denote the prevalence rate of never smokers and smokers, respectively; RR denotes the relative risk of mortality for smokers compared to never smokers; the subscript i is for disease category, r is for rural or urban district, s is for gender, and a is for age, which is classified into two groups: ages 35–64 and ages 65+.

Data Source

The primary data used in this paper were drawn from the third and fourth waves of the NHSS conducted by the Ministry of Health in China in 2003 and 2008, respectively. The surveys used standardized questionnaires to collect individual's information including age, gender, education, employment status, disease histories, health risk behaviors, healthcare utilization and expenditures for disease-specific outpatient visits and self-medication (not surveyed in 2008) in the two weeks before the date of interview, as well as disease-specific inpatient hospitalizations and number of inpatient days in the 12 months before the date of interview. Multi-stage stratified random sampling procedures and methods were used to select the samples. A total of 193,689 and 177,501 respondents aged 0 and above were sampled in 2003 and 2008, respectively.

Smoking prevalence rates by rural/urban district, gender, and age came from the 2003 and 2008 NHSS in which all respondents aged 15+ were asked about their smoking status. We divided respondents into never smokers and smokers (including current and former smokers). We did not separate current smokers from former smokers because the relative risks (RRs) of mortality needed to calculate SAFs have not been estimated separately for former and current smokers in China. (Note that former smokers accounted for only a small proportion of ever smokers in China, ranging from 10.1% in 1998 to 8.6% in 2008. See more details in the Results section.) The RRs of the mortality for smoking came from a recent study by Gu *et al.*; [18] population data and disease-specific mortality rates in 2003 and 2008 were taken from China's Health Statistical Yearbook; [19, 20] per-capita family income, used to measure earnings for the indirect cost of mortality, was from the China Statistical Yearbook [21, 22]. Life expectancy in 2003 came from the 2000 China Life Tables reported by the World Health Organization (WHO), while the 2008 life expectancy was from WHO's 2008 China Life Tables [23].

Direct Costs

Direct costs include all the healthcare expenditures for treating smoking-related diseases. Three types of healthcare expenditures were available in the 2003 NHSS data: inpatient hospitalizations, outpatient visits, and self-medication. However, only two types of healthcare expenditures were available in the 2008 NHSS data: inpatient hospitalizations and outpatient visits. The smoking-attributable expenditure (SAE) for each subgroup stratified by disease category, urban/rural district, gender, and age was estimated by multiplying the SAF by the corresponding total healthcare expenditures according to the following formula:

$$\text{SAE}_{\text{irsa}} = \big[\text{PH}_{\text{irsa}} \times \text{QH}_{\text{irsa}} + \text{PV}_{\text{irsa}} \times \text{QV}_{\text{irsa}} \times 26$$
$$+ \text{PM}_{\text{irsa}} \times \text{QM}_{\text{irsa}} \times 26\big] \times \text{POP}_{\text{rsa}} \times \text{SAF}_{\text{irsa}} \qquad (2)$$

where PH is the average expenditure per inpatient hospitalization; QH is the average number of hospitalizations per person in 12 months; PV is the average expenditure per outpatient visit; QV is the average number of outpatient visits per person in two weeks; PM is the average medication expenditures per person with positive self-medication expenditures in two weeks; QM is the proportion of persons with positive self-medication expenditures in two weeks; POP is the population in 2003 or 2008. The definition of subscripts is the same as with equation 1.

To assure that the self-reported health expenditures are a good proxy for actual expenditures, we applied an adjustment factor, which was determined as follows. First, we estimated the average per capita health expenditure for each disease category by urban/rural district, gender, and age from the 2003 and 2008 NHSS data. Second, we multiplied this number by the population in 2003 and in 2008 for each subgroup and added all the expenditures across all subgroups to derive the estimated national health expenditures in 2003 and 2008. Finally, we calculated the adjustment factor by dividing the estimated national health expenditures by the official figures of national health expenditures [24] and then applied this adjustment factor to the estimated average expenditures from the NHHS data. The adjustment factor was 1.22 for 2003 and 1.30 for 2008.

Indirect Morbidity Costs

Smoking-attributable indirect morbidity costs (SAI) include transportation, nutritious supplemental food, and caregiver costs during the inpatient hospitalizations and outpatient visits due to treating smoking-related diseases, and the value of lost productivity caused by smoking-related illness. We measured lost productivity by the number of days absent from work. Because days lost from work were not asked in the 2003 and 2008 NHSS, we used inpatient hospitalization days as a proxy. The formula to estimate the SAI is as follows:

$$\begin{aligned} SAI_{irsa} = \big[&PHI_{irsa} \times QH_{irsa} + PVI_{irsa} \times QV_{irsa} \times 26 \\ &+ IDAY_{irsa} \times E_{rsa} \times Y_r \big] \times POP_{rsa} \times SAF_{irsa} \end{aligned} \qquad (3)$$

where PHI is the average expenditures for transportation, nutritious supplemental food, and caregivers per inpatient hospitalization; PVI is the average expenditure for transportation per outpatient visit; IDAY is the average number of annual inpatient days due to treating disease "i" per employed person; E is the proportion of the total population currently employed; and Y is daily earnings measured by per-capita family income in 2003 or 2008. Other notations are the same as in equations 1 and 2.

Indirect Mortality Costs

The indirect mortality costs were estimated by four steps. First, the number of smoking-attributable deaths (SAD) was estimated by multiplying the SAF by total number of deaths for each 5-year age group from age 35–39 to age 85+ by population subgroups. Second, the number of smoking-attributable years of potential life lost (SAYPLL) was estimated by the product of the SAD and the number of years of life expectancy remaining at the age of death by population subgroups. Third, the present value of forgone lifetime earnings (PVLE) was estimated by 5-year age groups based on a human capital approach developed by Max and colleagues [25, 26]. A discount rate of 3% was used to convert a stream of earnings into its current worth. To consider the potential growth of future earnings, we assumed an annual productivity growth rate of 10%, approximately the average growth rate of GDP in China between 2003 and 2008. Fourth, smoking-attributable mortality cost (SAMC) was estimated by the product of the SAD and PVLE. The formulas we used to estimate SAD, SAYPLL, PVLE, and SAMC by disease category, urban/rural district, gender, and age group are:

$$SAD_{irsa} = \left[DRATE_{irsa} \times POP_{rsa} \right] \times SAE_{irsa} \tag{4}$$

$$SAYPLL_{irsa} = SAD_{irsa} \times LE_{sa} \tag{5}$$

$$PVLE_{rsa} = \sum_{m=a}^{\max a} \left[SURV_{rsa}(m) \right] \left[Y_r \times E_{rs}(m) \right]$$

$$\times (1 + g)^{m-a} / (1 + V)^{m-a} \tag{6}$$

$$SAMC_{irsa} = SAD_{irsa} \times PVLE_{rsa} \tag{7}$$

where DRATE is death rate per 100,000 persons, LE is average number of years of life expectancy remaining at the age of death, SURV(m) is the probability that a person will survive to age m, maxa is the maximum 5-year age group (e.g., age 85+), Y is per-capita family income, E(m) is the proportion of the population of age m that is employed in the labor market, g is the growth rate of labor productivity, V is the discount rate, a is the age at death, and other notations are the same as in equations 1 and 2.

Comparison of Cost Estimates Across Years

All the cost estimates are expressed in 2008 constant US dollars. We first estimated the costs of smoking for 2003 and 2008 in terms of nominal Chinese Yuan. Then, the estimated 2003 costs of smoking were converted into 2008 constant Chinese Yuan by multiplying by 1.19 based on the Consumer Price Index (CPI) for 2003 and 2008 in China [21]. Finally, we applied the 2008 exchange rate of 6.9451 Yuan against US$ to convert the costs into 2008 US dollars. Since the 2000 costs of smoking were estimated in terms of 2000 US dollars, [10] we first converted them back into 2000 Chinese Yuan by multiplying by the 2000 exchange rate of 8.2784. Then, following the process described above, we multiplied them by the ratio of the 2008 CPI to the 2000 CPI in China (1.20) and the 2008 exchange rate of 6.9451.

RESULTS

In the last decade, China has experienced a rapid growth in the adult population aged 35+ and a significant increase in internal migration from rural to urban areas. The population of persons aged 35+ increased from 515.6 million in 2000 to 601.4 million (17% increase) in 2003 and to 724.2 million (40% increase) in 2008. In 2000, 63.8% of these adults lived in rural areas. That percentage dropped to 59.5% in 2003 and decreased further to 54.5% in 2008 [21, 22, 27]. Because of the change in population mix, it is important to examine how smoking prevalence trends and patterns changed over the period, Table 1 shows prevalence rates of ever smokers among adults aged 35+ by urban/rural district, gender, age, and survey year according to the NHSS data. The prevalence rates for ever smokers decreased moderately from 38.0%

Table 1: Ever Smoking Prevalence Rate (%) Among Adults Aged 35 and Older in China, by Urban/Rural District, Gender, Age, and Year

	2003	2008
Total	33.1	31.4
Female in rural	4.6	4.5
35~64	4.0	3.9
65+	7.8	7.2
Female in urban	5.3	4.7
35~64	3.5	3.7
65+	10.7	7.4
Male in rural	64.0	61.3
35~64	65.2	62.9
65+	58.0	54.0
Male in urban	56.1	53.0
35~64	60.3	58.1
65+	42.3	37.1

(which included 34.5% as current smokers and 3.5% as former smokers) in 1998 [10] to 33.1% (30.6% as current smokers and 2.5% as former smokers) in 2003 to 31.4% (28.7% as current smokers and 2.7% as former smokers) in 2008. The quit rate, expressed as a proportion of ever smokers who are former smokers, remained low, decreasing slightly from 10.1% in 1998 to 8.6% in 2008. Male smoking rates remained much higher than female smoking rates. For males, rural smoking rates were higher than urban smoking rates; the opposite was found for females. Smoking prevalence rates in 2008 were lower than in 2003 across all subgroups by urban/rural, gender, and age except for females aged 35–64 in urban areas.

Table 2 shows the relative risks of mortality used in this study and the estimated SAFs calculated from equation (1). The relative risks of mortality for smokers were slightly higher for females and were highest for cancer. The SAFs were much smaller for females than males because smoking rates for

Table 2: Disease-specific Relative Risk of Mortality for Ever Smokers Smoking-attributable Fractions (SAFs) in China, 2008, by Disease, Urban/Rural District, Gender, and Age for Adults Aged 35 and Older

			SAF(%)							
	RR*		Urban				Rural			
			Male		Female		Male		Female	
	Male	Female	35~64	65+	35~64	65+	35~64	65+	35~64	65+
2003										
Respiratory diseases	1.14	1.43	7.78	5.59	1.48	4.40	8.36	7.51	1.69	3.25
Cardio-vascular diseases	1.17	1.21	9.30	6.71	0.73	2.20	9.98	8.98	0.83	1.61
Cancer	1.55	1.62	24.91	18.87	2.12	6.22	26.39	24.18	2.42	4.61
2008										
Respiratory diseases	1.14	1.43	7.52	4.93	1.57	3.08	8.09	7.03	1.65	3.00
Cardio-vascular diseases	1.17	1.21	8.99	5.93	0.77	1.53	9.66	8.41	0.81	1.49
Cancer	1.55	1.62	24.22	16.95	2.24	4.39	25.7	22.9	2.36	4.27

*Source: Gu and Kelly *et al.* (2009) [18].

Table 3:   Number of Deaths and Years of Potential
Life Lost (YPLLs) Attributable to Smoking in China,
2008, by Urban/Rural District, Gender, Age, and
Disease Among Adults Aged 35 and Older

	Deaths	YPLLs
Male	495,053	7,785,011
Female	57,227	720,609
35~64	215,994	5,340,087
65+	336,286	3,165,533
Urban	154,745	2,396,498
Rural	397,535	6,109,122
Respiratory diseases	61,514	628,559
Cardiovascular diseases	147,792	1,882,707
Cancer	342,974	5,994,354
Total	552,280	8,505,620

females were much lower than for males. The SAFs in 2008 were lower than in 2003 except for females aged 35–64 in urban areas, a pattern mimicking that of smoking prevalence. Among the three disease categories, cancer showed the highest SAFs for both males and females in 2008, ranging from a high of 25.7% for rural males aged 35–64 to a low of 2.2% for urban females aged 35–64.

As shown in Table 3, in 2008, 552,280 deaths in China were attributed to smoking — 495,053 males and 57,227 females; 154,745 in urban areas and 397,535 in rural areas — accounting for 8.9% of all deaths. By underlying cause of death, the majority of all smoking-attributable premature deaths were due to cancer (62%), followed by cardiovascular diseases (27%) and respiratory diseases (11%). The total number of smoking-attributable years of potential life lost (YPLLs) was 8.5 million person-years so the average years of life lost per death was 15.4 years. While cancer caused 62% of smoking-attributable deaths, it accounted for 92% of the total smoking-attributable YPLLs probably because most smokers who died of cancer died at a younger age than smokers who died from other causes. The death and YPLLs were calculated from equation (4) and (5).

Table 4 shows the economic costs of smoking in 2008 by component of costs, gender, age, urban/rural district, and disease. The total economic

Table 4: Economic Costs of Smoking in China, 2008, by Component of Costs, Urban/Rural District, Gender, Age, and Disease for Adults of Age 35 and Older Unit: US$1000

	Direct Medical Cost			Indirect Cost						
				Indirect Morbidity Cost						
	Outpatient	Inpatient	Subtotal	Transportation and Caregivers	Absence from Work	Indirect Mortality Cost	Subtotal	Total		
Male	4,054,280	1,483,162	5,537,442	332,547	226,410	20,778,363	21,337,320	26,874,762		
Female	485,233	178,926	664,159	50,741	35,842	1,226,432	1,313,015	1,977,174		
35~64	2,453,321	985,257	3,438,578	252,682	218,471	20,202,605	20,673,758	24,112,336		
65+	2,086,192	676,831	2,763,023	130,606	43,781	1,802,190	1,976,577	4,739,600		
Urban	1,999,408	835,647	2,835,055	136,550	71,405	10,471,987	10,679,942	13,514,997		
Rural	2,540,105	826,441	3,366,546	246,738	190,847	11,532,808	11,970,393	15,336,939		
Respiratory diseases	761,862	172,042	933,904	77,121	113,266	833,698	1,024,085	1,957,989		
Cardiovascular diseases	2,177,300	729,573	2,906,873	170,861	111,062	4,007,352	4,289,275	7,196,148		
Cancer	1,600,351	760,473	2,360,824	135,306	37,924	17,163,745	17,336,975	19,697,799		
Total	4,539,513	1,662,088	6,201,601	383,288	262,252	22,004,795	22,650,335	28,851,936		

Exchange rate of the Chinese Yuan against US$ = 6.9451 in 2008 based on China Statistical Yearbook, 2009 [21].

costs of smoking in 2008 amounted to $28.9 billion: $6.2 billion (21.5%) in direct costs, $22.0 billion (76.1%) in indirect mortality costs, and $0.7 billion (2.4%) in indirect morbidity costs.

The $28.9 billion of total economic costs in 2008 represented 0.7% of China's GDP ($4,360.7 billion). According to the NHSS data, the economic cost of smoking on average was $21.70 for each Chinese (= $28.9 billion/1.33 billion of total population) or $127.30 per smoker for the 227 million current smokers aged 35 and older in 2008. Because China's total consumption of cigarettes in 2008 was 2,139 billion sticks (107.0 billion packs), [22] the total economic costs of smoking averaged $0.27 per pack, about 8.1% of the 2006 average retail price of Class A cigarettes per pack in China (26.7 Yuan or $3.35) and about 43% of the price of Class B cigarettes per pack (5.0 Yuan or $0.63) [28]. A larger share of the total economic costs of smoking was borne by males than females ($26.9 billion versus $2.0 billion) and by the middle-aged group than the older age group ($24.1 billion versus $4.7 billion). Cancer comprised the highest proportion of the total economic costs in 2008: $19.7 billion (68.2%), followed by cardiovascular diseases at $7.2 billion (24.9%) and respiratory diseases at $2.0 billion (6.9%).

The $6.2 billion of direct costs of smoking in 2008 accounted for 3.0% of China's national healthcare expenditures ($209.3 billion): 73% of the direct costs of smoking were spent on outpatient visits while 27% was spent on inpatient care.

8-Year Comparison

Table 5 shows that the absolute number of smoking-attributable deaths decreased from 2000 to 2003 and then continued to fall from 2003 to 2008. This drop in deaths was due mainly to the declining trends in smoking prevalence and the resulting decrease in SAFs during the 8-year period (see Tables 1–2 in this paper and Table 1 by Sung et al. (2006) [10]). For example, the SAF for cancer among urban males aged 35–64 declined from 28.9% in 2000 to 24.9% in 2003 and declined again to 24.2% in 2008. Compared to 2000, the smoking-attributable YPLLs in 2003 decreased by 15.8% because of the declining SAFs and the use of the same life expectancy data for both 2000 and 2003. However, the YPLLs rose between 2003 and 2008 even though the number of smoking-attributable deaths fell. This resulted because updated life expectancy data were available in 2008, [23] and they revealed a substantial

Table 5: Comparison of Smoking-attributable Deaths, Years of Potential Life Lost, and Economic Costs in 2000, 2003, and 2008

	2000	2003	2008	Percentage Change(%) 2000–2003	Percentage Change(%) 2000–2008
Mortality	688,512	574,107	552,280	−16.62	−19.79
YPLL	9,699,251	8,162,771	8,505,620	−15.84	−12.31
Direct costs	2,439,796	4,198,072	6,201,601	72.07	154.19
Outpatient visits	1,285,832	2,472,829	4,539,513	92.31	253.04
Inpatient hospitalization	936,051	651,875	1,662,088	−30.36	77.56
Self-medication	217,913	1,073,368	—	392.57	—
Indirect costs	4,761,023	12,871,102	22,650,335	170.34	375.75
Transportation and caregivers	175,169	149,348	383,288	−14.74	118.81
Absence from work	387,006	159,392	262,252	−58.81	−32.24
Mortality	4,198,848	12,562,362	22,004,795	199.19	424.07
Total	7,200,819	17,069,174	28,851,936	137.04	300.68

Exchange rate of the Chinese Yuan against US$ = 6.9451 in 2008 based on China Statistical Yearbook, 2009 [21].

increase in life expectancy among Chinese from 68.9 years for males and 73.0 years for females in 2000 to 72.1 years for males and 75.7 years for females in 2008.

Compared to 2000, the total economic costs of smoking rose by 137% in 2003 and 300.7% in 2008. From 2000 to 2003, the direct costs of smoking costs increased by 72%. Smoking-attributable inpatient hospitalization costs fell by 30%, perhaps because of the decrease in the hospitalization rate [11]. The smoking-attributable self-medication costs grew dramatically by 393% during this period. From 2000 to 2008, the direct costs of smoking increased by 154%, and smoking-attributable outpatient costs alone increased by 253%. Compared to 2000, indirect mortality costs of smoking increased by 199% in 2003 and by 424% in 2008; the smoking-attributable costs of absence from work were lower in both 2003 and 2008 probably because they were based on inpatient days instead of work loss days; the smoking-attributable costs for transportation and caregivers decreased slightly by 15% in 2003 but increased by 119% in 2008.

DISCUSSION

The total economic cost of smoking for 2008 in China was $28.9 billion, accounting for 0.7% of China's GDP and averaging $127.30 per smoker. Among the different components of smoking-attributable costs, mortality costs ranked first, followed by outpatient expenditures. Alarmingly, 93.1% of the total economic cost of smoking in China was borne by males in 2008 because of their high smoking prevalence rate. Our results indicate that smoking is not only a matter of public health concern, which deserves attention, but it also has already exerted a huge financial burden on the Chinese economy.

The direct costs of smoking in 2008 accounted for 3.0% of total national health care expenditures in China [21]. This proportion is similar to that estimated by Sung *et al.* (3.1%) [10]. Yet it is lower than the 4.3% in Vietnam, [29] 4.7% in India, [30] and 6~8% in the United States [31]. Our estimates for the total direct and indirect costs of smoking are very likely underestimated for several reasons.

First, our estimation for the costs attributable to smoking considered only the three major categories of smoking-related diseases. Smoking increases the risk of many other diseases such as hip fractures, gum diseases, nasal irritation, nuclear cataract and Graves' ophthalmopathy, reproductive and erectile dysfunction problems, and peptic ulcers [5]. The omission of these diseases certainly results in underestimating the true costs of smoking.

Second, this study did not consider the economic burden from passive smoking. A recent study in Hong Kong found that this burden represented 23% of the total medical costs of active and passive smoking [32]. In China, 540 million persons (aged 0 and older) are exposed to passive smoking [33]. Thus, ignoring the economic impact of passive smoking underestimates the direct costs of smoking.

Third, the RR (relative risk of mortality) was an important element in estimating the SAF. The bigger this value, the larger the SAF (smoking-attributable fraction). In this study, we used the RRs from a prospective cohort study in a nationally representative sample of Chinese adults aged 40+ with baseline data collected in 1991 and follow-up evaluation collected in 1999–2000 [18]. The study's RR estimates for China were lower than those of other countries. For example, their RR estimate of lung cancer mortality in China for ever smokers relative to never smokers was 2.44 for males and 2.76 for females [18]. According to an American study, the corresponding RR estimate was 23.26 for current male smokers, 8.7 for former male smokers, 12.69 for current female smokers, and 4.53 for former female smokers [34]. The RR estimate of respiratory diseases in China for ever smokers was 1.14 for males and 1.43 for females; however, a recent nationally representative case-control study of smoking and mortality conducted in India estimated the corresponding RR in India to be 2.1 for males and 3.1 for females [35].

Fourth, it is particularly worth noting that according to the 2008 NHSS data, 10.6% of Chinese aged 15 and older who reported having medical conditions in the previous two weeks did not get any treatment in China in 2008, and 27.2% of Chinese who reported a need for hospitalization during the previous year were not hospitalized [27]. The corresponding figures in 2003 were 13.1% and 29.6%, respectively. These data suggest that smoking-attributable diseases might have occurred among these two groups of people, yet they did not utilize healthcare services. If this potential demand for healthcare services is transformed into real demand, smoking will impose a greater healthcare burden on the economy.

Finally, this study did not consider days lost from work by relatives or informal caregivers who took care of the patients with smoking-related illness. In addition, due to the lack of work loss data, the productivity losses due to smoking-caused disability other than inpatient hospitalization days were not considered. Therefore, the actual indirect morbidity costs of smoking-attributable diseases should be higher than our estimates (see more discussion below).

Our 2003 and 2008 cost estimates can be directly compared to the 2000 costs estimated by Sung *et al.* [10] because both studies employed the same methodologies with two exceptions. First, our study used the RRs of mortality for smoking from a more recent study by Gu *et al.* (2009) [10] rather than from Liu *et al.* (1998) [36] as did Sung *et al.* If we had used the RRs data from Liu *et al.*, [36] then the total economic cost of smoking in China in 2008 would be $23.0 billion instead of $28.9 billion, direct healthcare costs would be $5.2 billion instead of $6.2 billion, and indirect morbidity and mortality costs would be $17.8 billion instead of $22.7 billion. Therefore, part of the increases in the costs of smoking between 2000 and 2008 was due to the use of more recent RRs data, which we believe better capture the impact of smoking during the study period. Second, this study measured lost productivity by inpatient days as a proxy for work loss days [10] because the latter variable was not asked in the 2003 and 2008 NHSS. According to a published report based on the second wave of the NHSS data, [37] the annual average inpatient days in China were lower than the annual average work loss days by 23% for cancer, 41% for cardiovascular diseases, and 60% for respiratory diseases. Therefore, our estimates for the 2003 and 2008 indirect costs of absence from work could be underestimates by at least 23%.

During the eight years from 2000 to 2008, smoking-attributable deaths decreased by 20%, but the mortality costs of smoking increased by 836%. The decrease in smoking-attributable deaths is a consequence of the reduced smoking prevalence and the resultant decrease in SAFs plus the reduced mortality rates for cancer, cardiovascular, and respiratory diseases [19, 20]. The increase in the mortality costs of smoking is due mainly to the substantial increase in labor costs measured by per capita family income, which doubled from 2000 to 2003 and quadrupled from 2000 to 2008 in urban districts and which increased by 10% from 2000 to 2003 and by 96% from 2000 to 2008 in rural districts [21, 22, 27]. The direct healthcare cost of smoking rose by 72% from 2000 to 2003 and by 154% from 2000 to 2008. This large increase occurred because China's national healthcare expenditures increased dramatically from 550 billion Yuan in 2000 to 784 billion Yuan in 2003 and 1,454 billion Yuan in 2008 (all expressed in 2008 constant Yuan), as a result of introducing hightech medical equipment, the rising prices of healthcare services, and the growth of the population aged 35+ [20]. The increases in per capita family income and national healthcare expenditures were contributors to the prominent growth of China's national economy during the last decade.

In summary, our results indicate that smoking imposes a substantial burden on Chinese society. We found that the economic burden of smoking increased substantially during the eight years from 2000 to 2008 and that the increase was due largely to China's rapid economic growth. If China's economy continues to grow, the economic costs of smoking in the future will escalate if smoking prevalence cannot be substantially reduced. In the era of fast economic growth in China, stronger tobacco control measures must be taken without delay. Although currently 7.0% of China's central government total revenue is generated from tobacco profit and taxes ($64.8 billion in 2008), this share has been shrinking in recent years [21]. Tobacco's contribution is expected to shrink more in the future with the growth in the national economy, high tech, and other industries as observed in developed countries. Regardless, policymakers should understand the negative impact of cigarette smoking on China's financial burden. Raising tobacco excise taxes has been proven as the most effective tobacco control measure to reduce tobacco use while raising government tax revenue [38]. China currently levies a 76.7% tax rate at the producer level, equivalent to a 43.4% tax rate at the retail level, [39] which is a relatively low rate compared to cigarette tax rates around the world, the median of which is about 60% [40]. This relatively low rate suggests ample room for tobacco tax increases in China especially for Class B cigarettes. Moreover, our results show that the total economic burden of smoking averaged $0.27 per pack (or 43% of the Class B cigarette retail price per pack in 2006). As explained above, because our cost estimates are underestimated, the true burden of smoking could be much higher than $0.27 per pack. Therefore, the Chinese government should raise tobacco taxes on the retail price of Class B cigarettes without delay. Such an increase will help to offset the health-related financial losses to the society due to smoking and reduce cigarette smoking and its huge health-related financial burden. From an equity perspective, part of the tax revenues raised should be used to help remaining smokers quit and obtain health care for treating smoking-related illnesses that they may already have.

ACKNOWLEDGMENTS

This study was sponsored by the China Medical Board News (CMB) and partially supported by the US National Institutes of Health, Fogarty International Center, grant no. R01-TW05938. The authors are grateful to Section Chief Ling Xu and Master Yaoguang Zhang, Centre of Health Statistics and Information, Ministry of Health, China, for their advice and support during the process of data analysis.

What this paper adds

This paper provides an update on the economic costs attributable to smoking in China.

REFERENCES

1. Chinese Center for Disease Control and Prevention. [accessed 12 September 2010] Global adult tobacco survey (GATS) fact sheet China. 2010. http://www. cdc.gov/tobacco/global/gats/countries/wpr/fact_sheets/china/2010/index.htm

2. Doll R, Hill AB. A study of the aetiology of carcinoma of the lung. *BMJ*. 1952; 4797:1271–86. [PubMed: 12997741]

3. Gao YT, McLaughlin JK, Blot WJ, *et al*. Risk factors for esophageal cancer in Shanghai, China. I. Role of cigarette smoking and alcohol drinking. International Journal of Cancer. 2006; 58:192–96.

4. Proia NK, Paszkiewicz GM, Nasca MA, *et al*. Smoking and smokeless tobacco-associated human buccal cell mutations and their association with oral cancer — A review. Cancer Epidemiol Biomarkers Prev. 2006; 15:1061–77. [PubMed: 16775162]

5. US Department of Health and Human Services. The health consequences of smoking: a report of the Surgeon General. Atlanta, Georgia: US Department of Health and Human Services, Centers for Disease Control and Prevention, National Center for Chronic Disease Prevention and Health Promotion, Office on Smoking and Health; 2004.

6. Niu SR, Yang GH, Chen ZM, *et al*. Emerging tobacco hazards in China. 2. Early mortality results from a prospective study. BMJ. 1998; 317:1423–4. [PubMed: 9822394]

7. Hu TW, Mao Z, Ong M, *et al*. China at the crossroads: the economics of tobacco and health. Tob Control. 2006; 15(Suppl I):i37–41. [PubMed: 16723674]

8. Chen J, Cao JW, Chen Y, *et al*. Evaluation of medical cost lost due to smoking in Chinese cities. Biomed Environ Sci. 1995; 8:335–41. [PubMed: 8719175]

9. Jin SG, Lu BY, Yan DY, *et al*. An evaluation of smoking-induced health costs in China (1988–1989). Biomed Environ Sci. 1995; 8:342–9. [PubMed: 8719176]

10. Sung HY, Wang L, Jin S, *et al*. Economic burden of smoking in China, 2000. Tob Control. 2006; 15(Suppl I):i5-i11. [PubMed: 16723677]

11. Ministry of Health. People's Republic of China. An Analysis Report of National Health Services Survey in 2008. Beijing: Peking Union Medical College Press; 2010.

12. Kang HY, Kim HJ, Park TK, *et al*. Economic burden of smoking in Korea. Tob Control. 2003; 12:37–44. [PubMed: 12612360]

13. Levin ML. The occurrence of lung cancer in man. Acta Unio Int Contra Cancrum. 1953; 9:531–41. [PubMed: 13124110]

14. Lilienfeld, AM.; Lilienfeld, DE. Foundations of Epidemiology. 3. New York: Oxford University Press; 1994. p. 202.

15. Shultz, JM. SAMMEC: Smoking-attributable mortality, morbidity, and economic costs (computer software and documentation). Minneapolis: Minnesota Department of Health, Center for Nonsmoking and Health; 1986.

16. U.S. Centers for Disease Control and Prevention (CDC). Current trends state-specific estimates of smoking-attributable mortality and years of potential life lost — United States. 1985 MMWR. 1988; 37:689–93. [PubMed: 3141767]

17. Shultz JM, Novotny TE, Rice DP. Quantifying the disease impact of cigarette smoking with SAMMEC II software. Public Health Rep. 1991; 106:326–33. [PubMed: 1905056]

18. Gu DF, Kelly TN, Wu XG, *et al*. Mortality attributable to smoking in China. N Engl J Med. 2009; 360:150–9. [PubMed: 19129528]

19. Ministry of Health, People's Republic of China. China's Health Statistical Yearbook 2004. Beijing: Ministry of Health; 2004.

20. Ministry of Health, People's Republic of China. China's Health Statistical Yearbook 2009. Beijing: Ministry of Health; 2009.

21. National Bureau of Statistics of China. China Statistical Yearbook 2009. Beijing: China Statistics Press; 2009.

22. National Bureau of Statistics of China. China Statistical Yearbook 2004. Beijing: China Statistics Press; 2004.

23. World Health Organization. [accessed 5 May 2010] Life tables for WHO member states in 2000 and in 2008. http://apps.who.int/whosis/database/life_tables/life_tables.cfm

24. China National Health Economic Institute. China National Health Accounts Digest. Beijing: China Statistics Press; 2009.

25. Max W, Rice DP, Sung HY, *et al.* The economic burden of smoking in California. Tob Control. 2004; 13:264–67. [PubMed: 15333882]

26. Max, W.; Rice, DP.; Sung, H-Y., *et al.* Valuing human life: estimating the present value of lifetime earnings. University of California; San Francisco: Institute for Health and Aging; 2004b. http:// repositories.cdlib.org/ctcre/esarm/PVLE2000 [accessed 16 Oct 2009]

27. National Bureau of Statistics of China. China Statistical Yearbook 2001. Beijing: China Statistics Press; 2001.

28. Hu AG, Hu LL. Tobacco control policy analysis in China: taxes and price. Jia Ge Li Lun Yu Shi Jian. 2009; 11:27–8. (in Chinese).

29. Ross H, Trung DV, Phu VX. The costs of smoking in Vietnam: the case of inpatient care. Tob Control. 2007; 16:405–9. [PubMed: 18048618]

30. John RM, Sung HY, Max W. Economic cost of tobacco use in India, 2004. Tob Control. 2009; 18:138–43. [PubMed: 19131453]

31. Warner KE, Hodgson TA, Carroll CE. Medical costs of smoking in the United States: estimates, their validity, and their implications. Tob Control. 1999; 8:290–300. [PubMed: 10599574]

32. McGhee SM, Ho LM, Lapsley HM, *et al.* Cost of tobacco-related diseases, including passive smoking, in Hong Kong. Tob Control 2006; 15:125–30. [PubMed: 16565461]

33. Yang GH, Ma JM, Liu N, *et al.* Smoking and passive smoking in China, 2002. Zhonghua Liu Xing Bing Xue Za Zhi. 2005; 26:77–83. (in Chinese). [PubMed: 15921604]

34. Centers for Disease Control and Prevention. Adult SAMMEC: smoking-attributable mortality, morbidity, and economic costs (online software). Atlanta, GA: Centers for Disease Control and Prevention; 2010. https://apps.nccd.cdc.gov/sammec/edit_risk_data.asp [accessed 7 May 2010]

35. Jha P, Jacob B, Gajalakshmi V, *et al.* A nationally representative case-control study of smoking and death in India. N Engl J Med. 2008; 358:1137–47. [PubMed: 18272886]

36. Liu BQ, Peto R, Chen ZM, *et al.* Emerging tobacco hazards in China: 1. Retrospective proportional mortality study of one million deaths. BMJ. 1998; 317:1411–22. [PubMed: 9822393]

37. Ministry of Health, People's Republic of China. Research on National Health Services — an analysis report of the Second National Health Services Survey in 1998. Beijing: National Center for Health Information and Statistics; 1999.

38. Hu, TW.; Mao, ZZ.; Shi, J., *et al.* Tobacco taxation and its potential impact in China. Paris: International Union Against Tuberculosis and Lung Disease; 2008.

39. Hu TW, Mao ZZ, Shi J. Recent tobacco tax rate adjustment and its potential impact on tobacco control in China. Tob Control. 2010; 19:80–2. [PubMed: 19850552]

40. Mackay, J.; Eriksen, M. The tobacco atlas. Geneva: World Health Organization; 2002. p. 94–5.

Secondhand Smoke Exposure at Home in Rural China*

Tingting Yao, Hai-Yen Sung, Zhengzhong Mao,
Teh-wei Hu and Wendy Max

ABSTRACT

Purpose This study estimated secondhand smoke (SHS) exposure at home among nonsmoking children (age 0–18) and adults (age ≥ 19) in rural China, and examined associated socio-demographic factors.

Methods A total of 5,442 nonsmokers (including 1,456 children and 3,986 adults) living in six rural areas in China were interviewed in person. The standardized questionnaire obtained information on their demographic characteristics and SHS exposure at home. Differences in SHS exposure were assessed by use of the chi-squared test. Logistic regression analysis was used to examine the associated factors.

Results Occurrence of SHS exposure at home among nonsmoking children and adults was 68.0 and 59.3%, respectively. Logistic regression analysis found that children living in households with married, low-education, and low-income heads of household, and those who resided in the Qinghai province of China were more likely to be exposed to SHS. Among adults, those who were female, aged 19–34, single, low-education, and low-income, and those who lived in Qinghai province were more likely to be exposed to SHS at home.

Conclusions Our findings of substantial SHS exposure at home in rural China emphasize the importance of implementing interventions to reduce SHS exposure among this population.

*Published in *Cancer Causes Control*, 2012; 23: 109–115. DOI: 10.1007/s10552-012-9900-6.

INTRODUCTION

China has the largest number of smokers of any country in the world. In 2010, prevalence of smoking among adults in China was 28.1%: 52.9% for men and 2.4% for women [1]. More than 556 million nonsmoking adults in China were exposed to secondhand smoke (SHS) [2]. Adult current smoking prevalence in China decreased from 31.1% in 2002 to 28.1% in 2010 [1, 3]. However, there was an overall increase in the number of adults exposed to SHS during this period (from 540 million to 556 million) [2, 3]. In rural areas, the prevalence of SHS exposure greatly increased from 54.0% in 2002 to 74.2% in 2010 [2, 3].

Studies in developed countries have revealed that SHS exposure is associated with negative effects on health including respiratory illness, cancer, and heart disease [4, 5]. There are very few studies examining SHS exposure and its effect on health or economic burden in China. In one study, Gan and colleagues estimated that exposure to SHS was associated with more than 22,000 deaths from lung cancer and 33,800 ischemic heart disease deaths in China in 2002, equivalent to half a million years of healthy life lost [6]. In another study, Li and colleagues estimated the total economic costs attributable to SHS exposure in China at 29.4 billion Yuan (US$ 4.3 billion) in 2005 [7] (exchange rate: 1US$ = 7.0 Yuan).

In China, the term *rural areas* is usually used to refer to areas other than cities, and these areas are often characterized by relatively low population density and socioeconomic status [8]. According to the 2009 China Statistical Yearbook [9], 721.3 million Chinese people lived in rural areas in 2008, accounting for over half (54.3%) of China's population. Compared with the urban population, the rural population in China had much lower per capita net annual income (15,781 Yuan vs. 4,761 Yuan, equal to approximately US$2,254 vs. US$680). Furthermore, whereas the number of people completing only elementary school education or less was 16.5% in the urban population, it was fully 38.2% in the rural population [9]. It is common that a household consists of multiple generations in rural China; most residents are living at home and working in the family business. A previous study reported that SHS exposure in rural China was higher than that in urban areas (74.2 vs. 70.5% in 2010) [2]. Another study found that the prevalence of SHS exposure at home (82.0%) is greater than in public places (67.0%) and workplaces (35.0%) in China [3]. Therefore, persons living in rural China are more likely to be exposed to SHS at home than those living in urban settings. Several studies have been conducted on SHS exposure in work places and public places in China [10–12]. However, little research has focused on SHS exposure and associated factors in the home environment in rural China.

The objective of this study was to examine SHS exposure at home and its associated sociodemographic factors in rural China. The study examined SHS exposure for two age groups: children (age 0–18) and adults (age ≥19). A number of terms are used to describe exposure to other people's smoking, including environmental tobacco smoke (ETS), sidestream smoke, and passive smoking. The term "SHS" was used in this study. This paper addressed two questions:

(1) What is the prevalence of SHS exposure at home among children and adults in rural China?
(2) What are the factors associated with exposure to SHS at home in rural China?

This information will enable policymakers to better understand the prevalence of SHS exposure in rural China, and will provide evidence of the circumstances and individual characteristics that lead to the greatest likelihood of being exposed.

METHODS

Data Source

We used data from the 2008 China National Rural Household Survey (NRHS). The NRHS is a survey of Chinese rural households conducted by the China National Health Development Research Center in 2008 in six of China's provinces (or province-level municipalities): Qinghai (northwest), Anhui (east), Hubei (middle), Yunnan (west), Jiangsu (east), and Chongqing (southwest, a province-level municipality). These provinces cover approximately one sixth of the entire area of China and account for 21% of China's population [9]. Using multistage stratified random sampling methods, three rural villages were randomly selected in each province. The NRHS contains data from 18 villages from widely scattered geographic locations, indicating that the data cover a large variety of rural areas in China.

Study Design and Sample

A total of 1,801 households participated in this survey. Using a standardized questionnaire, a face-to-face interview was conducted with the head of household, who reported all the information including smoking behavior in the NRHS questionnaire on behalf of every household member. The questionnaire consisted of three sections:

(1) Sociodemographic characteristics (including age, gender, marital status, education, family net income in previous year, and region).
(2) Smoking status. The smoking status section contained two questions: "Have you ever smoked?", and "Did you smoke cigarettes in the previous 30 days". If the answer to the second question was "yes", the participant was classified as a current smoker.
(3) The relationship with the head of household, which was used to define whether a participant lived with current smokers.

Although smokers may also suffer harmful health effects from SHS exposure, it is hard to separate the effects from those due to active smoking. Thus, our analysis of SHS exposure focused only on nonsmokers, who were not "current smokers" as defined above. Eight children and 1,545 adults were classified as current smokers and hence were excluded. In this study, a person was defined as being exposed to SHS at home if they lived with at least one current smoker. After further excluding two respondents with missing smoking status and sociodemographic factor data, a total of 5,442 nonsmokers (1,456 children and 3,986 adults) were included in the final study sample.

Sociodemographic Measures

Sociodemographic characteristics include age, gender, marital status, education, income, and region. Marital status was classified as single, married, and divorced or widowed. Education was categorized as low education (less than high school), middle education (high school), and high education (more than high school). The per capita net income in the previous year was the ratio of family net income in the previous year to the number of household members. We then classified per capita net income in the previous year into three categories based on the cut-offs for the rural area from the 2009 China Statistic Yearbook [9]: low income (<2,218 Yuan, equal to US$317), middle income (2,218–5,066 Yuan, equal to US$317–723) and high income (>5,066 Yuan, equal to US$724). For children, their marital status, education, and income were defined by the status of the head of household.

Statistical Analysis

All analyses were conducted with STATA, version 11.0 (Stata, College Station, TX, USA). Differences in SHS exposure by sociodemographic characteristics were tested by use of chi-squared statistics. We used two logistic regression models to analyze factors associated with SHS exposure at home in rural China — one for children and one for adults. Adjusted odds ratios (AOR) and the corresponding 95% confidence intervals (CI) were computed to assess the strength of association. For the two logistic regression analyses, the dependent variables were whether children were exposed to SHS at home, and whether adults were exposed to SHS at home: 1 represented exposure and 0 represented non-exposure. The independent variables included all the sociodemographic characteristics. A two-tailed p value of <0.05 was considered statistically significant.

RESULTS

Sociodemographic Characteristics

Among children (Table 1), half (52.4%) were male, 60.4% aged 0–12, and 65.4% lived in a household headed by a married person. Most of them lived in households headed by someone with low education (75.6%) and low-middle income (81.9%). Two-thirds (67.7%) of nonsmoking adults were female (Table 2); one third (33.7%) were aged 19–34; and most were married (78.7%) and lived in low education (87.3%) and low-middle income (75.5%) households. As shown in Tables 1 and 2, the sample of nonsmoking adults was distributed quite evenly across regions, and the largest sample size for children was from Yunnan (23.8%).

SHS Exposure by Sociodemographic Characteristics

The prevalence of SHS exposure at home in rural China was 61.3% for all ages — 68.0% for children and 59.3% for adults. The chi-squared test (Tables 1 and 2) in univariate analysis showed that all the sociodemographic

Table 1: Prevalence of Exposure of Nonsmoking Children to SHS, by Sociodemographic Characteristics; Rural China, 2008

Demographic Characteristic	Children ($n = 1,456$)		
	Total % (n)	SHS Exposure %	p Value
Gender			
Male	52.4 (763)	65.4	.030*
Female	47.6 (693)	70.7	
Age			
0–12	60.4 (879)	70.2	.025*
13–18	39.6 (577)	64.6	
Marital status (of head of household)			
Single	32.9 (478)	62.4	.001*
Married	65.4 (953)	71.2	
Divorced and widowed	1.7 (25)	52.0	
Education (of head of household)			
Low (<high school)	75.6 (1,100)	68.5	.010*
Middle (high school)	22.7 (331)	68.3	
High (>high school)	1.7 (25)	40.0	
Per capita net income (of head of household)			
Low	38.4 (559)	71.1	.047*
Middle	43.5 (633)	67.4	
High	18.1 (2,674)	62.9	
Region			
Hubei	17.3 (252)	5,408	<.001*
Qinghai	18.4 (269)	78.1	
Yunnan	23.8 (346)	66.6	
Chongqing	12.1 (177)	67.2	
Anhui	18.4 (268)	73.2	
Jiangsu	9.9 (144)	66.7	
Total		68.0	

*$p < 0.05$ (2-tailed, chi-squared test).

characteristics examined in this study were significantly related to SHS exposure at home.

Factors Associated with SHS Exposure

In the logistic regression analysis, we found that all the sociodemographic factors considered in this study were statistically significantly associated with SHS exposure at home for both children (Table 3) and adults (Table 4),

Table 2: Prevalence of Exposure of Nonsmoking Adults to SHS, by Sociodemographic Characteristics; Rural China, 2008

Demographic Characteristic	Adults ($n = 3,986$)		
	Total % (n)	SHS Exposure %	p Value
Gender			
Male	32.3 (1,286)	41.8	<.001*
Female	67.7 (2,700)	67.7	
Age			
19–34	33.7 (1,345)	67.3	<.001*
35–64	53.8 (2,144)	54.8	
≥65	12.5 (497)	57.5	
Marital status			
Single	13.4 (537)	67.7	<.001*
Married	78.7 (3,135)	58.5	
Divorced and widowed	7.9 (314)	52.9	
Education			
Low (<high school)	87.3 (3,479)	59.9	.026*
Middle (high school)	9.6 (381)	53.0	
High (>high school)	3.2 (126)	52.7	
Per capita net income			
Low	31.9 (1,270)	61.8	.047*
Middle	43.6 (1,739)	59.0	
High	24.5 (977)	56.7	
Region			
Hubei	20.0 (797)	47.6	<.001*
Qinghai	17.5 (698)	67.5	
Yunnan	15.0 (597)	67.2	
Chongqing	15.8 (630)	57.8	
Anhui	17.4 (693)	60.5	
Jiangsu	14.3 (571)	58.0	
Total		59.3	

*$p < 0.05$ (2-tailed, chi-squared test).

except that gender and age were not significant for children. For children, SHS exposure at home was more likely:

— among those living in households headed by a married person than among those living in households headed by a single person;
— among those living in households headed by a low education person than among those living in households headed by high education person;

Table 3: Adjusted Odds Ratios from Logistic Regression Model Predicting SHS Exposure at Home for Children

Demographic Characteristic	Children ($n = 1,456$)	
	Adjusted Odds Ratio	95% CI
Gender		
Male	Reference	
Female	1.24	.99–1.56
Age		
0–12	Reference	
13–18	.94	.70–1.28
Marital status (of head of household)		
Single	Reference	
Married	1.40*	1.01–1.92
Divorced and widowed	.62	.27–1.45
Education (of head of household)		
Low (<high school)	2.69*	1.17–6.20
Middle (high school)	3.08	1.31–7.27
High (>high school)	Reference	
Per capita net income (of head of household)		
Low	1.51*	1.08–2.11
Middle	1.21	.89–1.66
High	Reference	
Region		
Hubei	Reference	
Qinghai	2.54*	1.54–3.25
Yunnan	2.23*	1.72–3.75
Chongqing	1.66*	1.10–2.49
Anhui	1.48*	1.04–2.09
Jiangsu	1.53	1.00–2.37

*$p < 0.05$ (2-tailed).

— among those living in low income households than among those living in high income households; and

— among those residing in Qinghai, Yunnan, Chongqing, or Anhui province than among those residing in Hubei province.

For adults, females, single people, and young adults aged 19–34 were more likely to be exposed to SHS exposure at home than males, married people, and adults aged 65 and older. Similar to children, adults who had low education,

Table 4: Adjusted Odds Ratios from Logistic Regression Model Predicting SHS Exposure at Home for Adults

Demographic Characteristic	Adults ($n = 3,986$)	
	Adjusted Odds Ratio	95% CI
Gender		
Male	Reference	
Female	3.34*	2.88–3.86
Age		
19–34	1.34*	1.03–1.75
35–64	.77*	.62–.97
≥65	Reference	
Marital status		
Single	1.68*	1.30–2.18
Married	Reference	
Divorced and widowed	.64	.48–.83
Education		
Low (<high school)	1.56*	1.01–2.41
Middle (high school)	1.21*	0.71–1.76
High (>high school)	Reference	
Per capita net income		
Low	1.23*	1.02–1.48
Middle	1.08	.91–1.28
High	Reference	
Region		
Hubei	Reference	
Qinghai	2.13*	1.70–2.66
Yunnan	1.86*	1.48–2.35
Chongqing	1.42*	1.14–1.77
Anhui	1.48*	1.19–1.84
Jiangsu	1.36*	1.08–1.70

*$p < 0.05$ (2-tailed).

low income, and who lived in Qinghai or other provinces were more likely to be exposed to SHS than those with high education, high income, and from Hubei.

DISCUSSION

The findings of this study indicate very high prevalence (61.3%) of SHS exposure at home in rural China in 2008, with prevalence significantly higher among children than adults (68.0 vs. 59.3%). We found SHS exposure at home among adults in rural China (59.3%) was higher than previously reported by Wang *et al.* (48.3%) [13]. Our findings of substantial SHS exposure at home in rural China, coupled with the fact that 54.3% of China's population lives in rural areas, emphasize the importance of implementing tobacco control intervention to reduce SHS exposure among this population.

Previous studies have shown that health education is critical to improving people's knowledge about the harm of SHS and attitudes towards SHS exposure [14–16]. For children, school-based education which adds appropriate content on SHS-related matters, for example information about the harm of SHS exposure and skills in persuading smokers not smoke in front of them, into school curricula could have a positive effect on reducing SHS exposure. For adults, it has been shown that health-education programs can increase knowledge about the harm of SHS exposure, move attitudes towards stronger disapproval, and increase the likelihood of taking assertive action when exposed to SHS in the family [17].

Also, smoke-free law in public places could be another effective way of reducing SHS at home in rural China. A recent study conducted in the US found that strong clean indoor air laws in public places and work places are associated with large increases in voluntary smoke-free-home policies in homes both with and without smokers [18]. China passed a smoke-free rule in all public indoor spaces (including restaurants, bars, Internet cafes, and public transport) on May 1, 2011, but violators can be still seen everywhere because of lack of enforcement. Thus, smoke-free laws plus strict enforcement are needed in China.

In addition, we found that the rural area in Qinghai province had the highest SHS exposure, consistent with the 2007 China Tobacco Control Report [19]. Qinghai is located in the northwest part of China, with an economy amongst the smallest in all provinces of China. Its nominal GDP for 2009 was just 108.1 billion RMB (US$15.8 billion) and contributes approximately 0.3% of national GDP. Per capita GDP was 19,407 RMB (US$2,841), the second lowest in China [20]. This emphasizes the importance of implementing tobacco-control programs in these less-developed areas in China.

Furthermore, we found that women and low socio-economic status (SES) groups (low education and income) were more likely to be exposed to SHS.

This is consistent with a previous study in China, which showed that females and those with low education level were more likely to be exposed to household SHS, because most women are housewives in the county area of China and thus spend most of their time at home [13]. Several studies have shown that SHS exposure increases the risk of premature death among women and children [21], breast cancer among women [22], and asthma among children [23]. However, there is not yet enough awareness of this significant public health issue among women in rural China. In rural areas of China, most women work at home in family businesses. Thus, our findings indicate the importance of creating a smoke-free home environment for low SES children and women, as they may more often live in households with smokers where smoking occurs.

This study revealed that single adults were more likely to be exposed to SHS at home than married adults. This may be explained by the fact that more than half (56.6%) of the single adults from the 2008 NRHS survey were aged 19–34. It is common for three generations to live together in rural China. Because smoking prevalence among the older generation aged ≥35 was higher than among the young adult generation aged 19–34 (31.1 vs. 20.6%, according to 2008 NRHS data), the young adult generation is more likely to live with current smokers than the older generation, which results in more SHS exposure at home. This phenomenon is consistent with the findings that children were more likely than adults to be exposed to SHS at home. However, more studies are needed to further examine the association between marital status and SHS exposure at home.

This study has several limitations. First, only one representative per family was interviewed, and he/she reported smoking status information for all the other family members. This response by proxy could potentially cause underestimation of the prevalence of SHS exposure. This might explain the different level of adult SHS exposure at home in rural China found in the 2010 Global Adults Tobacco Survey in China compared with this study (67.3 vs. 59.3%), given that the former interviewed individuals directly. Second, because of the design of the NRHS questionnaire, SHS at home was measured by whether or not a nonsmoker lives with at least one current smoker at home, which could lead to overestimation of the prevalence of SHS exposure, because a smoking family member might not smoke inside the home and expose others to SHS. Ideal measures might be a question such as "How many days per week did a smoker smoke in front of you?" [13] or biomarker measures, for example hair and urine nicotine [24, 25]. Unfortunately, this information is not available in this study. However, because many persons in rural areas lack knowledge about SHS exposure, they may not be aware of the fact that smoking in front of nonsmokers exposes them to SHS. As a result, we believe that living with a current smoker is a good proxy for SHS exposure at home for rural China. Third, Chinese parents might not be willing to report that their children smoke, because smoking is not regarded as good behavior for women and children in China. This could lead to social desirability bias in which SHS exposure is underestimated because the numbers of smokers in a household is under-reported or children reported as exposed are, in fact, smokers. However, it is not clear what the effects on the estimates would be. Despite these limitations, this study indicates the potential need to develop a comprehensive intervention program for reducing SHS exposure at home in rural China.

In conclusion, this study documents high prevalence of SHS exposure at home among nonsmoking children and adults living in rural China. Given the large proportion of Chinese people who live in rural areas, there is great potential to reduce the harmful effects of tobacco exposure by designing intervention that reduce SHS exposure among this population.

ACKNOWLEDGMENTS

This study was conducted with support from the US National Institutes of Health, Fogarty International Center (grant R01 TW05938), the US National Cancer Institute (grant CA-113710), the Australia Government's Overseas Aid Program (HSS080020), the China-Australia Health and HIV/AIDS Facility, the Operational Research on Integration of NCMS and MA Rural Health Financing Schemes, the Sichuan University Scientific Research Foundation for Young Teachers, and the Flight Attendants Medical Research Institute (FAMRI). The authors would like to thank the China National Health Development Research Center for collection of the data, and members of the UCSF Writer's Task Force for their helpful comments and suggestions.

Conflict of Interest The authors declare that they have no conflict of interest.

REFERENCES

1. Chinese Center for Disease Control and Prevention (2010) Global adult tobacco survey (GATS) fact sheet China. http://www.cdc.gov/tobacco/global/gats/countries/wpr/fact_sheets/china/2010/index.htm. Accessed 25 March 2011.

2. Chinese Center for Disease Control and Prevention (2011) Tobacco control and China's future. http://www.notc.org.cn/n4772065/n5001162/40983.html. Accessed on March 29, 2011 (Chinese).

3. Yang GH, Ma JM, Liu N *et al.* (2005) Smoking and passive smoking in Chinese, 2002. Zhonghua Liu Xing Bing Xue Za Zhi 26:77–83 (Chinese).

4. U.S. Department of Health and Human Services (US DHHS) (2006) The health consequences of involuntary exposure to tobacco smoke: a report of the surgeon general — executive summary. U.S. Department of Health and Human Services, Centers for Disease Control and Prevention, Coordinating Center for Health Promotion, National Center for Chronic Disease Prevention and Health Promotion, Office on Smoking and Health.

5. California Environmental Protection Agency (CA EPA) (2005) Proposed Identification of environmental tobacco smoke as a toxic air contaminant. California Environmental Protection Agency, Office of Environmental Health Hazard Assessment: Sacramento, CA, US.

6. Gan Q, Smith KR, Hammond SK *et al.* (2007) Disease burden of adult lung cancer and ischaemic heart disease from passive tobacco smoking in China. Tob Control 16:417–422.

7. Li L, Chen QL, Jia RX *et al.* (2008) The smoking pattern and disease burden of tobacco use in China. Chin Health Econ 27(1):26–30.

8. Hou GB, Wang XC, Zhou F (2008) Comment on definition of peasant and village under PE building background of new village and division of peasants group. J Xiangnan Univ 29(5):108–111.

9. 3-1 Population and Its Composition, China Statistical Yearbook (2009) China Statistics Press.

10. Gan Q, Hammond SK, Jiang Y *et al.* (2008) Effectiveness of a smoke-free policy in lowering secondhand smoke concentrations in offices in China. J Occup Environ Med 50(5):570–575.

11. Zheng P, Li W, Chapman S *et al.* (2011) Workplace exposure to secondhand smoke and its association with respiratory symptoms — a cross-sectional study among workers in Shanghai. Tob Control 20(1):58–63.

12. Liu R, Hammond SK, Hyland A *et al.* (2011) Restaurant and bar owners' exposure to secondhand smoke and attitudes regarding smoking bans in five Chinese cities. Int J Environ Res Public Health 8(5):1520–1533.

13. Wang CP, Ma SJ, Xu XF *et al.* (2009) The prevalence of household second-hand smoke exposure and its correlated factors in six counties of China. Tob Control 18(2):121–126.

14. Koh HK, Alpert HR, Judge CM *et al.* (2010) Understanding worldwide youth attitudes towards smoke-free policies: an analysis of the Global Youth Tobacco Survey. Tob Control. doi: 10.1136/tc.2010.038885.

15. Morello P, Linetzky B, Kaplan J (2010) Knowledge, attitudes, and practices of Argentine pediatricians regarding second hand smoke exposure in children. Arch Argent Pediatr 108(4):318–324.

16. Guyer B, Ma S, Grason H *et al.* (2009) Early childhood health promotion and its life course health consequences. Acad Pediatr 9(3):142–149.e1-71.

17. Lee AH (2008) A pilot intervention for pregnant women in Sichuan, China on passive smoking. Patient Educ Couns 71(3):396–401.

18. Cheng KW, Glantz SA, Lightwood JM (2011) Association between smokefree laws and voluntary smokefree-home rules. Am J Prev Med 41(6):566–572.

19. 2007 China Tobacco Control Report (2007) Ministry of Health, PRC, Beijing, China.

20. http://www.thechinaperspective.com/topics/province/qinghai-province/

21. Wipfli H, Avila-Tang E, Navas-Acien A (2008) Secondhand smoke exposure among women and children: evidence from 31 countries. Am J Public Health 98:672–679.

22. Reynolds P, Goldberg D, Hurley S *et al.* (2009) Passive smoking and risk of breast cancer in the California teachers study. Cancer Epidemiol Biomarkers Prev 18(12):3389–3398.

23. Cinar N, Dede C, Cevahir R *et al.* (2010) Smoking status in parents of children hospitalized with a diagnosis of respiratory system disorders. Bosn J Basic Med Sci 10(4):319–322.

24. Hsieh SJ, Ware LB, Eisner MD *et al.* (2011) Biomarkers increase detection of active smoking and secondhand smoke exposure in critically ill patients. Crit Care Med 39(1): 40–45.

25. Kalkbrenner AE, Hornung RW, Bernert JT *et al.* (2010) Determinants of serum cotinine and hair cotinine as biomarkers of childhood secondhand smoke exposure. J Expo Sci Environ Epidemiol 20(7):615–624.

The Healthcare Costs of Secondhand Smoke Exposure in Rural China*

Tingting Yao, Hai-Yen Sung, Zhengzhong Mao,
Teh-wei Hu and Wendy Max

ABSTRACT

Objective The goal of this study was to assess the healthcare costs attributable to secondhand smoke (SHS) exposure among non-smoking adults (age ≥ 19) in rural China.

Methods We analysed data from the 2011 National Rural Household Survey which was conducted among adults in five provinces and one municipality in China (N=12 397). Respondents reported their smoking status, health conditions and healthcare expenditures. Relative risks were obtained from published sources. Healthcare costs included annual outpatient and inpatient hospitalisation expenditures for five SHS-related diseases: asthma, breast cancer (female only), heart disease, lung cancer and tuberculosis. SHS-attributable healthcare costs were estimated using a prevalence-based annual cost approach.

Findings The total healthcare costs of SHS exposure in rural China amounted to $1.2 billion in 2011, including $559 million for outpatient visits and $612.4 million for inpatient hospitalisations. The healthcare costs for women and men were $877.1 million and $294.3 million, respectively. Heart disease was the most costly condition for both women ($701.7 million) and men ($180.6 million). The total healthcare costs of SHS exposure in rural China accounted for 0.3% of China's national healthcare expenditures in 2011. Over one-fifth of the total healthcare costs of SHS exposure

*Published in *Tob Control*, 2014; 0:1–6. doi: 10.1136/tobaccocontrol-2014-051621.

in rural China were paid by health insurance. The out-of-pocket expenditures per person accounted for almost half (47%) of their daily income.

Conclusions The adverse health effects of SHS exposure result in a large economic burden in China. Tobacco control policies that reduce SHS exposure could have an impact on reducing healthcare costs in China.

INTRODUCTION

China is the largest producer and consumer of tobacco in the world. According to the 2010 Global Adult Tobacco Survey, 301 million Chinese adults were current smokers, and the prevalence of smoking among adults in China was 52.9% for men and 2.4% for women in 2010.[1] In addition, a report from the Chinese Center for Disease Control and Prevention indicates that over 556 million adults were exposed to secondhand smoke (SHS) in China in 2010,[2] a number that was greater than the number of current smokers.

China's adult smoking prevalence has decreased recently, dropping from 31.1% in 2002[2] to 28.1% in 2010.[1] However, exposure to SHS in China did not decline in the past decade.[2] In rural areas, SHS exposure among those aged 15 years and above increased substantially from 54% in 2002 to 74.2% in 2010.[2,3] A recent study found that 68% of children and 67.7% of women living in rural areas were exposed to SHS at home in 2008.[4]

SHS exposure has been linked to several illnesses, including respiratory diseases and other adverse health effects in children, and lung cancer and heart disease in adults.[5,6] The health effects of SHS exposure could result in excess economic costs. A few studies have estimated the economic costs of SHS exposure in China. Leung *et al.*[7] examined the impact and economic costs associated with SHS exposure among infants in Hong Kong with non-smoking mothers. They found that postnatal exposure to SHS at home was linked to higher rates of hospitalisations for any illness compared with unexposed infants (OR=1.1), leading to 662 extra hospitalisations and $0.9 million excess inpatient costs in 1997. Gan *et al.*[8] estimated the disease burden of SHS exposure among Chinese adults aged 30 years or above and found that SHS exposure was responsible for the loss of nearly 230 000 years of healthy life from lung cancer, and more than one-quarter of a million years of healthy life from ischaemic heart disease. Li *et al.*[9] estimated that the total cost of SHS exposure in China was ¥14.5 billion (US$2.1 billion) in 2000, and ¥29.4

billion (US$4.3 billion) in 2005. No study to date has analysed the healthcare costs attributable to SHS exposure in rural China.

Since persons living in rural China often have lower income levels than urban dwellers, they may suffer a heavier economic burden from SHS exposure. Therefore, estimates of the health-related costs attributable to SHS exposure in rural China are needed to understand the economic impact of SHS exposure, and to motivate policymakers to implement smoke-free and other policies to reduce the health and economic toll. Accordingly, the objective of this study is to estimate the healthcare costs attributable to SHS exposure for non-smoking adults (age ≥ 19) in rural China.

METHODS

We used a prevalence-based, disease-specific approach to estimate SHS-attributable healthcare costs.

Data Sources

All analyses in this study were conducted using data from the 2011 *National Rural Household Survey* (*NRHS*). The NRHS is a nationally representative face-to-face survey of Chinese rural households conducted by the China National Health Development Center in 2011 in five provinces (Qinghai, Anhui, Hubei, Yunnan, Jiangsu) and one municipality (Chongqing) in China. These provinces and municipality cover about one-sixth of the geographic area of China with locations around the country, covering a range of rural areas in China. In the five provinces, three rural villages were randomly selected based on different income levels (high, middle and low). In Chongqing, two districts were randomly selected, and three rural villages were then randomly selected in each district.

The head of each household was interviewed, and he/she also reported on behalf of all household members. The questionnaire consisted of three sections with 114 total questions. The following variables from the NRHS were used in our study: (1) gender; (2) smoking status (those who answered 'yes' to the question 'Did you smoke cigarettes in the previous 30 days?' were classified as a 'current smoker'); (3) SHS exposure — defined by whether a participant lived with a current smoker or not; (4) chronic conditions in the past 12 months; (5) disease-specific costs for outpatient visits in the past month, and disease-specific costs for inpatient hospitalisations in the past 12 months; and (6) how much of outpatient visits and inpatient visits was covered by health insurance.

Study sample

A total of 4249 households (including 13 933 adults aged 19+) were interviewed in 2011. After excluding respondents with missing information on gender, smoking status, chronic conditions and healthcare expenditures, a total of 12 397 adults were included in the final study sample.

Measures

SHS exposure

Our study focused on non-smokers, that is, those who reported not being current smokers. Though smokers may also suffer harmful health effects from SHS exposure, it is difficult to separate the effects from those due to active smoking. We defined *non-smokers who are exposed to SHS* as those non-smokers who live in a household with at least one current smoker.

SHS-related diseases

We included five SHS-related diseases for adults based on the 2006 Surgeon General's report[5] and the 2005 California Environmental Protection Agency (EPA) report.[6] These diseases are asthma, breast cancer (for females aged 19–50 years only), heart disease, lung cancer and tuberculosis (TB), as shown in Table 1. In the NRHS, respondents could report one to three diseases diagnosed by doctors. Interviewers then recorded these disease names in the data set. We considered respondents to have SHS-related diseases if they reported any of the five diseases just discussed.

Relative risks

The relative risk (RR) of a disease from SHS exposure among non-smokers is defined as the ratio of the disease rate for exposed non-smokers to the disease rate for unexposed non-smokers. The RRs of SHS-related diseases were obtained from published studies conducted in China except for asthma. Since RR estimates for asthma have not been published for the Chinese population,

Table 1:   Relative Risk of Secondhand Smoke (SHS)-related Diseases

SHS-related disease	ICD-9 code	Relative Risks (95% CI)		Country of Study	Source
		Female	Male		
Asthma	493	1.97 (1.19 to 3.25)	1.97 (1.19 to 3.25)	Finland	Jaakkola *et al.*[10]
Breast cancer (female)	174	1.60 (1.00 to 2.40)	NA	China	Shrubsole *et al.*[11]
Heart disease	410–414	1.24 (1.15 to 1.34)	1.22 (1.10 to 1.35)	China	He *et al.*[12,13]
Lung cancer	162	1.13 (1.05 to 1.21)	1.13 (1.05 to 1.21)	China	Zhao *et al.*[14]
TB	011	1.55 (1.01 to 2.40)	1.55 (1.01 to 2.40)	China	Dong *et al.*[15]

NA, not applicable; TB, tuberculosis.

we used the RR estimates from a Finnish study,[10] as cited in the California EPA report.[6] The RRs by disease and gender are shown in Table 1.

SHS-attributable fraction

A smoking-attributable fraction is commonly used for the estimation of health or economic burdens attributable to smoking, such as disease incidence, healthcare utilisation and healthcare expenditures. Similarly, the SHS-attributable fraction (SAF_{shs}) measures the proportion of health or economic burden in the specific population (e.g., non-smoking adults) that can be attributed to SHS exposure. In this study, the SAF_{shs} for each subgroup stratified by disease (i) and gender (j) was estimated using the standard epidemiological formula (1)[16]:

$$SAF_{shs,ij} = \left[P_{shs,j} \times (RR_{shs,ij} - 1) \right] / \left[P_{shs,j} \times (RR_{shs,ij} - 1) + 1 \right] \quad (1)$$

where P_{shs} is the prevalence (%) of SHS exposure among non-smokers and RR_{shs} the RR of illness for non-smokers who were exposed to SHS compared to those who were not exposed.

Healthcare Costs

In this study, healthcare costs include expenditures for outpatient visits and inpatient hospital stays. Outpatient visits included ambulatory care visits at outpatient departments of hospitals and doctor visits at clinics. Expenditures for prescribed medicine during the outpatient visits or inpatient stays were included in the respective outpatient or inpatient expenditure categories.

In the NRHS, respondents were asked to report (1) the average outpatient expenditures per month for each disease treated in the past 6 months, and (2) the disease name and total inpatient expenditures, including out-of-pocket payment and insurance payment, for the most recent hospitalisation stay during the past 12 months. The SHS-attributable healthcare costs (SAE_{shs}) among the rural population was estimated by disease (i) and gender (j) by multiplying the SAF by the total healthcare expenditures (THE) for the non-smoking rural population according to the following formula:

$$SAE_{shs,ij} = THE_{ij} \times SAF_{shs,ij}$$
$$= POP_j \times P_{NS,j} \times DRATE_{ij}$$
$$\times (INPX_{ij} + OUTX_{ij} \times 12) \times SAF_{shs,ij} \qquad (2)$$

where POP denotes the rural adult population aged ≥ 19; P_{NS} is the percentage of rural adults who were non-smokers; DRATE is the disease prevalence rate among non-smoking rural adults; INPX denotes the average annual inpatient expenditures per person among rural non-smoking adults who had that SHS-related disease; and OUTX denotes the average monthly outpatient expenditures per person among rural non-smoking adults who had that SHS-related disease. POP was obtained from the 2011 Statistical Yearbook,[17] while all other variables were estimated from the 2011 NRSH data.

Health Insurance Coverage

In the NRHS, respondents were asked to report the annual outpatient expenditures covered by health insurance for each disease treated in the past 6 months and the inpatient expenditures covered by health insurance for the most recent hospitalisation stay during the past 12 months. We first calculated the mean value of costs covered by health insurance for each disease and then applied them to formula (2) to get the costs covered by health insurance among total SHS-attributable costs.

Sensitivity Analysis

Three sensitivity analyses were conducted. The first one was performed based on the lower bound and upper bound of the 95% CIs of RR estimates in Table 1. The second one was performed using the RRs of SHS-related diseases estimated from US studies[5,6,18,19] except for asthma, because the US RR estimates for asthma were not available. The third one was performed by using published disease rates for the Chinese population.[20–22] This was carried out because the disease rates reported in the NRHS are lower than those generally published.

RESULTS

Number of Non-smoking Adults Living in Rural China

The final study sample of the 2011 NRHS had nearly equal numbers of men and women, as shown in Table 2. Women were much more likely to be non-smokers, and among non-smokers the prevalence of SHS exposure was 62.2% for women and 35% for men.

Number of Persons with SHS-related Diseases Among Non-smoking Adults in Rural China

Table 3 shows the number and disease rates of SHS-related diseases in rural China by gender, type of healthcare service used and disease. Outpatient visits and inpatient hospitalisation were most often reported by people with heart disease (especially women), followed by TB and asthma. There were no inpatient hospitalisations reported for lung cancer or breast cancer.

Table 2: Prevalence of Non-smoking and Number of Non-smoking Adults Living in Rural China, 2011

	Percentage of Adults Who are Non-smokers from NRHS	Number of Adults Living in Rural China in 2011* (Millions)	Number of Non-smoking Adults in Rural China (Million)
Female	97.8	245.04	239.65
Male	47.6	257.29	122.47

*Source: China Statistical Yearbook.[17]
NRHS, National Rural Household Survey.

Table 3: Disease Prevalence Rate and Number of Persons with Secondhand Smoke (SHS)-related Diseases Among Non-smoking Adults in Rural China, 2011

	Disease Rate* (%)			Number of Persons with SHS-related Diseases among Non-smoking Adults in Rural China (1000)[†]		
	Female (N=6139)	Male (N=2919)	Total	Female	Male	Total
Outpatient visits						
Asthma	0.15	0.17	0.15	359	208	551
Breast cancer (female)	0.03	NA	0.03	72	0	110
Heart disease	3.31	2.02	2.89	7932	2474	10612
Lung cancer	0.02	0.03	0.02	48	37	73
TB	0.11	0.27	0.17	264	331	624
Inpatient hospitalisations						
Asthma	0.03	0.10	0.06	72	122	220
Breast cancer (female)	0	NA	0	0	NA	0
Heart disease	0.83	0.69	0.78	1989	845	2864
Lung cancer	0	0	0	0	0	0
TB	0.03	0.14	0.07	72	171	257

*Data source: NRHS survey.
[†] Derived by multiplying 'Disease rate' (1st column in Table 3) and 'Number of non-smoking adults in rural China' (last column in Table 2).
NRHS, National Rural Household Survey; TB, tuberculosis.

SHS-Attributable Healthcare Costs among Non-smokers in Rural China

Table 4 shows the estimated SAF_{shs} by gender, disease and healthcare service type. The SAF_{shs} values for all diseases were larger for women than men. Asthma had the highest disease-specific SAF_{shs} for both women (0.38) and men (0.25), while lung cancer showed the lowest SAF_{shs} for both women (0.07) and men (0.04).

Table 4 also shows the healthcare costs of SHS exposure by gender, disease and healthcare service type estimated as the product of the total number of persons with SHS-related disease, the average annualised costs per person with the SHS-related disease, and the SAF_{shs}. The total healthcare costs of SHS exposure in rural China in 2011 amounted to $1.2 billion: $559 million

Table 4: Secondhand Smoke (SHS)-attributable Fraction (SAFshs) and SHS-attributable Healthcare Costs Among Non-smokers in Rural China, 2011

SHS-related Diseases	SAF$_{shs}$ Female	SAF$_{shs}$ Male	Average Annual Healthcare Cost per Person with the SHS-related Disease ($) Female	Male	Cost Attributable to SHS Exposure ($ Million)[†] Female	Male	Total SHS-Attributable Cost ($ Million)	Costs Covered by Health Insurance ($ Million)
Outpatient								
Asthma	0.38	0.25	246	183	33.3	9.7	42.9	2.2
Breast cancer	0.27	NA	2057	NA	40.2	NA	40.2	2.0
Heart disease	0.13	0.07	349	362	359.6	64.0	423.6	21.7
Lung cancer	0.07	0.04	38	952	0.1	1.5	1.7	0.1
TB	0.25	0.16	371	481	24.9	25.7	50.6	2.5
Subtotal					458.1	100.9	559.0	28.5
Inpatient								
Asthma	0.38	0.25	413	1037	11.2	32.2	43.4	14.7
Breast cancer	0.27	NA	0	NA	0.0	NA	0.0	0.0
Heart disease	0.13	0.07	1324	1930	342.1	116.6	458.7	156.7
Lung cancer	0.07	0.04	0	0	0.0	0.0	0.0	0.0
TB	0.25	0.16	3587	1611	65.7	44.6	110.3	37.6
Subtotal					419.0	193.4	612.4	209.2
Total					877.1	294.3	1171.4	237.7

[†]It equals the product of the number of persons with SHS-related diseases (last column of Table 3), average annualised cost per person with the SHS-related disease and the SAF$_{shs}$, according to equation (2).
US$1=¥6.3 (exchange rate in 2011).
NA, not applicable; TB, tuberculosis.

for outpatient visits and $612.4 million for inpatient hospitalisations. The total cost for women ($877.1 million) was almost three times as high as the cost for men ($294.3 million). For women, heart disease was the most costly disease ($701.7 million), followed by TB ($90.6 million), asthma ($44.5 million), breast cancer ($40.2 million) and lung cancer ($0.1 million). For men, the results showed a similar pattern: heart disease was the most costly disease ($180.6 million), followed by TB ($70.3 million), asthma ($41.9 million) and lung cancer ($1.5 million). About one-fifth of healthcare costs ($237.7 million) were covered by health insurance, including $28.5 millon for outpatient visits and $209.2 million for inpatient visits.

Sensitivity Analyses

Table 5 shows that the total healthcare costs of SHS exposure in rural China in 2011 ranged from $573.6 million to $1.7 billion using the upper and lower bounds of the RR estimates. Costs almost doubled ($2.1 billion) when using the RRs for the US population and slightly increased to $1.22 billion when using the published disease rates for the Chinese population.

DISCUSSION

Our findings indicate that SHS exposure in rural China imposes a large economic burden ($1.2 billion) on China, accounting for 0.02% of China's gross domestic profit ($6.7 trillion in 2011[17]) and 0.3% of the national healthcare expenditures in 2011 ($385 billion in 2011[17]). Given the total rural population of 650 million in 2011,[17] this amounted to $1.80 per person in China. Nearly three-quarters of the total healthcare cost of SHS exposure in rural China was for women because a majority of women are non-smokers who live with smokers. Over one-fifth of the total healthcare cost of SHS exposure in rural China was paid by health insurance. The out-of-pocket expenditures per person ($1.44) accounted for almost half (47%) of their daily income ($3.03) in rural China.

Our estimates most likely underestimated the economic burden of SHS exposure for several reasons. First, our calculation only included five SHS-related diseases for adults. Children are also vulnerable to SHS exposure and suffer from diseases that are related to SHS exposure including low birth weight,[6] middle ear disease[6] and attention deficit hyperactivity dis-order.[23] According to the SHS exposure rate for children (68%) in rural China,[4] we estimated that about 100.4 million children were exposed to SHS in rural China in 2011. Therefore, the total costs would be much higher if the costs of children's SHS exposure could be also included. Second, our study was limited to direct healthcare costs only. Future studies that include indirect morbidity and mortality costs attributable to SHS exposure are needed. Third, besides the home environment, people are also exposed to SHS in workplaces and public places. A recent report in 2010[2] found that 73% and 63% of Chinese were exposed to SHS in public places and workplaces, respectively. However, we were not able to separate the impact of SHS exposure at home from exposure in other settings. Fourth, our study is based on self-reported data and only the

Table 5: Sensitive Analyses of Secondhand Smoke (SHS)-attributable Healthcare Costs Among Non-smokers in Rural China, 2001

SHA-related Disease	From NRHS Cost Attributable to SHS Exposure ($ Million)	From Sensitivity Analysis 1		From Sensitivity Analysis 2			From Senditivity Analysis 3	
		Cost Attributable to SHS Exposure ($ Million) Lower Bound of RR	Cost Attributable to SHS Exposure ($ Million) Upper Bound of RR	Using the Relative Risk (95% CI) for US Population		Cost Attributable to SHS Exposure ($ Million)	Using Published Disease Rates for the Chinese Population (%)	Cost Attributable to SHS Exposure ($ Million)
				Female	Male			
Outpatient								
Asthma	42.9	11.7	68.4	1.97 (1.19 to 3.25)[10]	1.97 (1.19 to 3.25)[10]	42.9	0.16[19]	44.6
Breast cancer	40.2	0	68.8	1.68 (1.31 to 2.15)[6]	NA	44.0	0.21[20]	281.3
Heart disease	423.6	266.5	581.0	1.50 (1.04 to 1.60)[5]	1.50 (1.40 to 1.60)[5]	790.1	0.77[19]	108.1
Lung cancer	1.7	0.7	2.6	1.29 (1.04 to 1.60)[6]	1.29 (1.04 to 1.60)[6]	3.5	0.04[21]	2.3
TB	50.6	1.2	97.8	2.33 (1.97 to 2.75)[19]	2.33 (1.97 to 2.75)[19]	94.8	0.08[22]	25.7
Subtotal	559.0	280.1	818.6			975.3		462.0
Inpatient								
Asthma	43.4	11.1	73.3	1.97 (1.19, 3.25)[10]	1.97 (1.19 to 3.25)[10]	43.4	0.16[19]	111.1
Breast cancer	0.0	0	0	1.68 (1.31 to 2.15)[6]	NA	0.0	0.21[20]	0.0
Heart disease	458.7	279.9	637.7	1.50 (1.04 to 1.60)[5]	1.50 (1.04 to 1.60)[6]	867.6	0.77[19]	447.5
Lung cancer	0.0	0	0	1.29 (1.04 to 1.60)[6]	1.29 (1.04 to 1.60)[6]	0.0	0.04[21]	0.0
TB	110.3	2.6	210.9	2.33 (1.97 to 2.75)[18]	2.33 (1.97 to 2.75)[18]	204.5	0.08[22]	200.8
Subtotal	612.4	293.5	921.9			1115.5		759.3
Total	1171.4	573.6	1740.0			2090.8		1221.4

NA, not applicable; NRHS, National Rural Household Survey; RR, relative risk; TB, tuberculosis.

head of the household was interviewed, which may create recall bias. Fifth, the RRs we used were lower than those from western countries. For example, the RR of heart disease among men was 1.22 for the Chinese population compared to 1.50 for the US population.[5] The RR of TB was 1.55 for the Chinese population compared to 2.33 for the US population.[19] According to the sensitivity analysis which assumed the RRs for the US population, we found that the estimated total healthcare costs attributable to SHS in rural China would almost double from $1.2 billion to $2.1 billion if we used the US RRs, and the costs would then account for 0.6% of China's national healthcare expenditures in 2011. The higher RRs in the US population reflect a more mature epidemic of smoking, and suggest that risks of smoking-related disease in China may increase in the future. Sixth, very few cases of SHS-related diseases were reported in the NRHS, with the exception of heart disease. It is possible that these diseases were under-reported due to the lack of a formal diagnosis. Therefore, we conducted another sensitivity analysis using disease rates from published Chinese studies and found that the estimated SHS-attributable total healthcare costs in rural China increased to $1.22 billion. In addition, the rate of outpatient visits for heart disease in our study was much higher than that from a published Chinese study (2.89% vs 0.77%). This might be because the latter study included all of China and our study focuses only on rural areas. More studies are needed to address this. Finally, the RRs used in this study were based on findings from previous studies, which did not control for exposure to air pollution. This may cause an upward bias of our estimated SHS-attributable fractions and healthcare costs.

The study by Yang et al.[24] provided the most recent estimate of the total healthcare cost of active smoking in China at $6.2 billion in 2008, including $2.8 billion for urban areas and $3.4 billion for rural areas. Converting these estimates into 2011 dollars using the Consumer Price Index (105.9 in 2008 and 105.4 in 2011),[17] the healthcare cost of active smoking for rural China would be $3.38 billion. Therefore, our estimated healthcare cost attributable to SHS exposure was more than one-third of the cost of active smoking in rural areas. The ratio of SHS costs to active smoking costs in our study was higher than a study conducted in Hong Kong, which reported a ratio of 29%.[25] Our study demonstrates that the true impact of smoking on healthcare costs in rural areas would be one-third higher than the estimates by Yang et al.[24] when the burden of SHS exposure is included. Given that the majority of women and children are non-smokers and exposed to SHS in rural China, tobacco control interventions that reduce SHS exposure are needed.

This research serves as a starting point for a comprehensive assessment of the health and economic impact of SHS exposure in China. The findings provide useful evidence for policymakers who are developing interventions to reduce SHS exposure and increase public awareness in China.

What this paper adds

What is already known on this subject

- The secondhand smoke (SHS) exposure rate increased substantially in the past decade in China. SHS exposure has been linked to several illnesses.
- No study to date has analysed the healthcare costs attributable to SHS exposure in rural China.

What important gaps in knowledge exist on this topic

- This study is the first to estimate the healthcare costs of SHS exposure in rural China.

What this study adds

- We found that the healthcare costs of SHS exposure constitute a large economic burden to China.
- Our findings demonstrate the importance of implementation of tobacco control policies that reduce SHS exposure in rural China as a means of reducing healthcare costs.

ACKNOWLEDGEMENTS

The authors would like to thank the China National Health Development Research Center for their collection of data.

Contributors T-wH and ZM obtained funding to conduct the National Rural Household Survey and helped collect data. TY conducted all the data analyses and wrote the first draft of the manuscript. WM and H-YS helped design the analytical approach and the data analysis and contributed to the interpretation of the analytical results. All authors provided comments, assisted in revising the drafts and approved the final manuscript.

Funding This study was funded by grants from the US National Institutes of Health Fogarty International Center (grant R01 TW009295) and the National Cancer Institute; the Australia Government's Overseas Aid Program (HSS080020), the China-Australia Health and HIV/AIDS Facility, the Operational Research on Integration of NCMS and MA Rural Health Financing Schemes; the California Tobacco-Related Disease Research Program, Cornelius Hopper Diversity Award Supplement (20CA-0102); the University of California, San Francisco Dorothy Pechman Rice Postdoctoral Fellowship; and the US National Cancer Institute (grant CA-113710).

Competing Interests None.

Patient Consent Obtained.

Ethics Approval Ethics approval was obtained from the Office of Research Ethics at the China National Health Development Center.

Provenance and Peer Review Not commissioned; externally peer reviewed.

REFERENCES

1. Chinese Center for Disease Control and Prevention. Global adult tobacco survey (GATS) fact sheet China. 2010. http://www.who.int/tobacco/surveillance/en_tfi_china_gats_fact sheet_2010.pdf (accessed 4 Dec 2013).
2. Chinese Center for Disease Control and Prevention. Tobacco control and China's future. 2011. http://www.12320.gov.cn/fujian/1295424820703.pdf (accessed 4 Dec 2013 (Chinese)).
3. Yang G, Ma J, Liu N, *et al.* Smoking and passive smoking in China, 2002. *Zhonghua Liu Xing Bing Xue Za Zhi* 2005;26:77–83. (in Chinese).
4. Yao T, Sung HY, Mao Z, *et al.* Secondhand smoke exposure at home in rural China. *Cancer Causes Control* 2012;23:109–15.
5. US Department of Health and Human Services (USDHHS). The Health Consequences of Involuntary Exposure to Tobacco Smoke: a Report of the Surgeon General. USDHHS, Center for Disease Control and Prevention, Office of Smoking and Health, 2006.
6. California Environmental Protection Agency. *Proposed Identification of Environmental Tobacco Smoke as a Toxic Air Contaminant.* 2005. http://www.ocat.org/pdf/CALEPA_toxic_report.pdf (accessed 31 Dec 2013).

7. Leung GM, Ho LM, Lam TH. The economic burden of environmental tobacco smoke in the first year of life. *Arch Dis Child* 2003;88:767–71.

8. Gan Q, Smith KR, Hammond K, *et al.* Disease burden of adult lung cancer and ischaemic heart disease from passive tobacco smoking in China. *Tob Control* 2007;16:417–22.

9. Li L, Chen Q, Jia R, *et al.* The smoking pattern and disease burden of tobacco use in China. *Chinese Health Economics* 2008;27:26–30. (in Chinese).

10. Jaakkola MS, Piipari R, Jaakkola N, *et al.* Environmental tobacco smoke and adult-onset asthma: a population-based incident case-control study. *Am J Public Health* 2003;93:2055–60.

11. Shrubsole MJ, Gao YT, Dai Q, *et al.* Passive smoking and breast cancer risk among non-smoking Chinese women. *Int J Cancer* 2004;110:605–9.

12. He Y, Lam TH. A review on studies of smoking and coronary heart disease in China and Hong Kong. *Chin Med J* 1999;8:1123–8.

13. He Y. Women's passive smoking and coronary heart disease (in Chinese). *Chin J Prev Med* 1989;23:19–22.

14. Zhao H, Gu J, Xu H, *et al.* Meta-analysis of the relationship between passive smoking population in China and lung cancer (in Chinese). *Zhongguo Fei Ai Za Zhi* 2010;13:617–23.

15. Dong B, Ge N, Zhou Y. Smoking and alcohol consumption as risk factors of pulmonary tuberculosis in Chengdu: a matched case-control study. *Hua Xi Yi Ke Da Xue Xue Bao* 2001;32:104–6. (in Chinese).

16. Lillienfeld AM, Lillienfeld DE. *Foundations of epidemiology.* 3rd edn. New York: Oxford University Press, 1994.

17. China Statistics Bureau. *China Statistical Yearbook.* Beijing: China Statistics Bureau, 2012.

18. Bates MN, Khalakdina A, Pai M, *et al.* Risk of tuberculosis from exposure to tobacco smoke: a systematic review and meta-analysis. *Arch Intern Med* 2007;167:335–42.

19. Center for Health Statistics and Information, China Ministry of Health. An Analysis Report of National Health Services Survey in China, 2008:p33.

20. Yu ZG, Jia CX, Liu LY, *et al.* The prevalence and correlates of breast cancer among women in Eastern China. *PLoS ONE* 2012;7:e37784.

21. Chen W, Zheng R, Zhang S, *et al.* Lung cancer incidence and mortality in China, 2009. *Thoracic Cancer* 2013;4:102–8.

22. World Bank Report: Incidence of tuberculosis. http://data.worldbank.org/indicator/SH. TBS.INCD (accessed 23 Jan 2013).

23. Max W, Sung HY, Shi Y. Attention deficit hyperactivity disorder among children exposed to secondhand smoke: a logistic regression analysis of secondary data. *Int J Nurs Stud* 2013;50:797–806.

24. Yang L, Sung HY, Mao ZZ, *et al.* Economic costs attributable to smoking in China: update and an 8-year comparison, 2000–2008. *Tob Control* 2011;20:266–72.

25. McGhee SM, Ho LM, Lapsley HM, *et al.* Cost of tobacco-related diseases, including passive smoking, in Hong Kong. *Tob Control* 2006;15:125–30.

Section II
Demand for Cigarette Consumption

Chapter 5

Quantity, Quality, and Regional Price Variation of Cigarettes: Demand Analysis Based on a Household Survey in China*

Yuyu Chen and Weibo Xing

ABSTRACT

This paper investigates the price elasticity of cigarettes using an urban household survey in China. We find that cigarette price is an important determinant of smoking. In our two-part model, the overall price elasticity is −0.82. Nevertheless, tobacco demand is influenced by both price and quality. We net out the quality effect of tobacco demand to obtain standard price elasticities, which are between −0.70 and −0.35. In addition, when we estimate two demand systems of Chinese households, the estimated own-price elasticities of cigarettes are −0.57 and −0.81. These elasticities suggest that if the tobacco excise tax rate goes up, cigarette consumption will drop rapidly, and government revenue from the tobacco tax will increase.

*Published in *China Economic Review*, 2011; 22, 221–232. doi: 10.1016/j.chieco.2011.01.004.

INTRODUCTION

Numerous studies have examined the negative effects of tobacco consumption on society. Tobacco use is one of the critical preventable causes of premature death. About one million people die in China each year from smoking-related diseases, the largest number of such deaths in the world (Hu, Mao, Shi, & Chen, 2008). In addition, smoking causes many chronic diseases that damage people's productivity and increase smokers' health-related expenditures. Carefully calculated estimates are that the direct and indirect costs of smoking in 2000 were about five billion dollars in China (Sung, Wang, Jin, Hu, & Jiang, 2006). Finally, the consumption of tobacco products also creates a huge negative externality on non-smokers.

Hoping to improve the health of the population in China and reduce the economic cost of smoking, policymakers have become very interested in tobacco consumption interventions. One of the most advocated interventions is a tax on tobacco products that might reduce tobacco consumption and correct for the negative externality. Additionally, the tobacco tax might be a good tool for collecting fiscal revenue for governments that have weak fiscal positions. To design a reasonable tax on tobacco products, policymakers need exact knowledge of the parameters of demand for tobacco products, including price elasticity, income elasticity, and other parameters governing consumers' behavioral responses. These parameters must be estimated using reliable data sets and proper econometric techniques.

China has a large population of smokers. According to the 2002 National Smoking Prevalence Survey, about 350 million individuals were smokers at some point, and 300 million are current smokers (Young, Ma, Liu, & Zhou, 2005). Recognizing the importance of tobacco control, the Chinese government ratified the 1995 WHO Framework Convention on Tobacco Control (FCTC). Recently, studies have provided information about the amount of tobacco products consumers are willing to buy when tobacco prices change. In this study, we estimate the behavioral response parameters of tobacco demand in China using several methods including the two-part model, the Deaton model (1988, 1989, 1997), and demand systems for a nationally representative cross-sectional data set. This data set includes precise information about the quantity of and the expenditures made on tobacco consumed in China from 1999 to 2001. In particular, the Deaton model is used to estimate quality elasticity and own-price elasticity for tobacco consumption.

The Deaton model is based on the assumption of regional price variation.[1] This model can be used to resolve the issue of endogeneity caused by price. Regional price variation has not been used often in demand analysis because of the belief that in high-income countries where transport systems are highly developed and transport costs are relatively low, price does not vary much across locations. Even in the United States, however, considerable regional variation exists in cigarette prices due to the substantial variation in state and local taxes. In New York City, for example, the tax alone is $4.25 per pack of cigarettes ($2.75 in state taxes and an additional $1.50 in local taxes), while in South Carolina, the tax is only $0.07 (Smith, 2010). Deaton (1997) also showed that in India and Pakistan, the price of tobacco products varied from village to village. Mao and Hu (2008) have argued that although the excise tax on cigarettes is unified in China, significant price disparity exists across regions. The reason for this disparity is the more than one hundred brands of cigarettes in China, the prices of which may vary from less than one yuan to over one hundred yuan per pack.

In this paper, we rely on a household survey, the Urban Household Income and Expenditure Survey (UHIES), to examine the price elasticity of tobacco consumption in China's urban population during the period 1999–2001. To determine the robustness of the elasticities estimated using the two-part model and the Deaton model, we use demand system methods[2] (Stone's Analysis, 1954; Linearized Almost Ideal Demand System (LA/AIDS), Deaton & Muellbauer, 1980a) to estimate own- and cross-price elasticities of household consumption of 10 commodities (including tobacco). Furthermore, because our study yields several price elasticities for tobacco consumption in urban China, we also investigate the implications of a tax on tobacco consumption and calculate potential fiscal revenue in China using a simple micro-simulation method.

To our knowledge, this is the first time that this survey has been used to analyze tobacco consumption in Chinese households. This paper is also one of

---

[1] "Spatial price variation" is used in Deaton (1988). Because "spatial" has been associated recently with spatial economics and spatial econometrics, we use "regional price variation" here to indicate the price disparity across locations.

[2] Yen, Fang, and Shew-Jiuan (2004) used a translog demand system to estimate household food consumption in urban China. They found prices played important roles in food demand and there were obvious regional differences.

the few research efforts that consider the quality effect of tobacco consumption using Deaton's method. This method can resolve endogeneity issues ignored by some research in which unit value (expenditure divided by quantity) is used to measure price. Using two demand system methods, the sensitivity tests also increase the credibility of the results obtained using the Deaton model. According to the complexity of optimal tax policy maximizing a welfare function, we assume that policymakers use taxes to reduce the consumption of tobacco by correcting the social costs generated by tobacco consumption. In this paper, we posit several reasonable tobacco taxes and then do some simple simulations to evaluate the impact of each of these taxes on tobacco consumption and fiscal revenue.

This paper is organized as follows. Section 2 briefly reviews the literature related to tobacco consumption. Section 3 is a simplified model drawn mainly from Deaton (1997) and used to show how to estimate price elasticity using unit value. Section 4 describes the data set. In Section 5, we first estimate price elasticity using the two-part model and the Deaton model to identify the price elasticity of tobacco products. In this section, we also use the demand systems of Stone's Analysis and the AIDS model to determine the own- and cross-price elasticity of tobacco use in sensitivity tests. Section 6 discusses the impact of increasing taxes on tobacco consumption and fiscal revenue using the estimated price and income elasticities. The final section offers conclusions.

LITERATURE REVIEW: MODELING TOBACCO CONSUMPTION

Much of the literature concentrates on modeling tobacco demand and the effects of prices (or taxes) on tobacco consumption. Chaloupka and Warner (2000) have provided an excellent introduction to the main economic issues in tobacco studies, including the impact of price (or taxes), the demographic structure of the population of smokers (e.g., age, education, and race), advertising, and smoking regulations. The Economics of Tobacco Toolkits by the World Bank also provide a comprehensive and in-depth handbook on many tobacco issues. These toolkits provide a variety of methods for dealing with tobacco data and analyzing tobacco demand. They also provide information on designing and administering a tobacco tax and the impact of tobacco control on employment, equality, smuggling, and other tobacco-related issues.

Our study focuses mainly on estimates of the price elasticity of tobacco consumption in China. We begin by reviewing the literature on tobacco consumption or tobacco demand. Different tobacco demand models have been developed based on time-series data, cross-sectional data, and panel data. The basic models used are conventional demand models such as the linear, double-log, log-lin, and lin-log models (Wilkins, Yurekli, & Hu, 2007). In general, these models are static. Other studies use dynamic models such as the rational addictive demand model (Becker & Murphy, 1988) or employ some dynamic demand specifications (Baltagi, Griffin, & Xiong, 2000). These models are usually based on time-series data or panel data. For example, some applications of the rational addiction model in individual-level surveys find that U.S. men behave more myopically and are relatively more responsive to price than U.S. women.

Over the past several decades, tobacco consumption has increased rapidly in low-income countries. Chapman and Richardson (1990) first estimated the impact of tobacco taxes on the demand for tobacco products in developing countries. They estimated a price elasticity of −1.42 for cigarettes and −1.00 for other tobacco products. According to Tansel (1993), the average price elasticity for cigarettes in Turkey was −0.21 for the short term and −0.37 for the long term at that time. Sayginsoy and De Beyer (2002) have analyzed the demand for cigarettes in Bulgaria. The price elasticity reported in their study was −0.80.

Several recent studies have produced estimates of the price elasticity of tobacco demand in China. Mao, Yang, Ma, Samet, and Ceraso (2003) estimated the price elasticity of cigarettes in the population at large (−0.513) and at various income levels (at the poverty level, −1.906; low-income, −0.774; high-income, −0.507). Lance, Akin, Dow, and Loh (2004) examined cigarette demand in China and Russia using longitudinal micro-level household surveys. The price elasticities reported (0 to −0.15) are smaller than in other studies on Chinese consumers. Mao, Hu, and Yang (2005) used a log-linear model and two-part models to evaluate the demand for cigarettes. Based on national aggregate data and individual data from a national tobacco consumption survey, they found a price elasticity of demand of −0.154 and discovered that higher price elasticity is associated with the low-income group. Bishop, Liu, and Meng (2007) estimated cigarette price and income elasticity for urban Chinese individuals in 1995 and found an overall cigarette price elasticity of −0.5.

Some research has used data from surveys including information on smoking status by individual or by household to estimate price and income elasticity. These surveys usually use cross-sectional data. Two types of models are used with cross-sectional data: two-stage least squares estimation (2SLS) with instrumental variables (IV) and the two-part model first developed by Cragg (1971) and subsequently used in other studies. In particular, using the two-part model can help one avoid the problems found in typical logarithmic regression models in which the dependent variable is zero for non-smokers. In this model, probit or logit regression is first used to estimate a smoking participation equation. Then the ordinary least squares (OLS) is used to estimate smoking intensity. However, this model fails to consider the potential problem that occurs because different types or brands of cigarettes are available to consumers. Some cigarettes have filters and some do not; some are longer than others; and some are Marlboro and others are Honghe (a popular low-priced brand of cigarettes in China). These variations create problems in estimating price elasticity for cigarettes.

Econometric techniques exist for dealing with endogenous quality changes so that real price elasticity figures can be determined. Deaton (1988) developed a technique for estimating price elasticity using cross-sectional household surveys in contexts with regional price variation. The data from household surveys in many countries reflect household-level expenditures and quantities for various consumer goods, so this method has been used in studies that use household survey data from various countries to estimate price elasticity of demand (Crawford, Laisney, & Preston, 2003). Nicita (2004) used the Deaton model and found that alcohol and tobacco consumption in Mexico was associated with large price elasticity in general (at a level of -0.91). John (2005) examined the demand for a variety of tobacco products in India using Deaton's method and the resulting price elasticities of tobacco products ranged from -0.5 to -1.0.

In addition, the question of how to adjust tax policy to influence tobacco consumption is very important. A tax adjustment may both reduce tobacco consumption and increase fiscal revenue to cover the health costs that arise from smoking (Escario & Molina, 2004). Deaton (1997) has offered a standard method for analyzing how tax reform affects household welfare. Measures of welfare change based on net compensating variations have been used in other studies as well (Niimi, 2005). Pogue and Sgontz (1989) suggested that the tobacco tax has two opposing effects on social welfare — it reduces the consumer surplus of smokers and simultaneously lowers the social costs that smokers impose on society, e.g., lost days at work and medical costs.

THE MODEL

Unit Values and Choice of Quality

Household surveys often collect data on expenditures and physical quantity consumed by households by category (e.g., cigarettes or other commodities). Dividing expenditure by physical quantity yields unit value figures. Unit value is not the same as price. An endogeneity issue exists if quantities are regressed on unit values and quantity elasticity directly. For tobacco, consumption is affected not only by price but also by quality. A pack of Marlboros costs a great deal more than a pack of Honghe. With such factors in mind, in addition to choosing a quantity of items to purchase, consumers also choose brands and types. That is to say, they choose a product with a particular level of quality. Thus, unit value is different from market price, over which consumers have no control. In turn, high-quality[3] items (or a mixture with a relatively large share of high-quality items) will have higher unit values. Opportunities to vary quality (or to choose different brands and types) will tend to attenuate the price elasticity of quantity. As prices rise, an individual can lower quality, pay less per pack, and continue to smoke the same quantity of cigarettes. In an extreme case, quantity elasticity may be close to zero because consumer response may exist purely in relation to quality, in which case the quality elasticity should be high.[4] For policy purposes, it is also important to control for quality effects in determining quantity price elasticity because from the perspective of public health, quantity elasticity is the more important consideration.

Because the unit value is chosen by the consumer, any attempt to use those figures to explain the demand for tobacco will expose a study to the risk

[3] High-quality tobacco product here does not refer to tobacco products that are good for people's health or that cause less damage to people's health. We use the term high-quality to refer to those tobacco items that cost a higher price for reasons like popularity, brand effect, etc.

[4] Deaton (1997) pointed out that between localities, uniformly higher prices in region A relative to B may cause a reduction in quality in region A and result in a unit value relatively close to region B. The differences in quantity between region A and B will be attributed to a smaller change in unit elasticity, thus exaggerating the quantity elasticity.

of simultaneity bias. In particular, because wealthier households tend to buy high-quality tobacco products, unit value will be positively related to income or total outlay. This relationship results in a serious econometric problem.

The Quality Effect

To reflect the quality effect, we use the following specification:

$$\ln v = \alpha^1 + \beta^1 \ln x + \gamma Z + u^1 \tag{1}$$

where $\ln v$ is log unit value, $\ln x$ is log total expenditure, Z is a vector of variables related to household characteristics, and u^1 is an error item. Other household characteristics, such as household size, gender-age ratio, education, and occupation are used to explain quality choice. The quality choice model was first examined by Prais and Houthakker (1955) using a household survey from Britain.

Note that unit values are determined not only by the choice of quality but also by actual market prices. Therefore, we should include actual market prices on the right-hand side of Eq. (1). However, doing this is impossible because we do not have the data on actual market prices. Nevertheless, it is possible to estimate the coefficients in Eq. (1) consistently if we assume that market price does not vary within clusters or neighborhoods. If this assumption holds, then we can estimate Eq. (1) with full clusters or neighborhood dummies. Under Deaton's (1997) assumption of regional price variation, we can estimate Eq. (1) to get β^1, which represents quality elasticity. This is the important parameter used to estimate our price elasticity below.

The Choice of Quality and Quantity

Households must be geographically clustered within the data set. Clustering is very important because it means that households within each cluster can be assumed to have approximately the same price options available. In this study, a cluster is defined as a set of households in the same area (a province in our study).

Another assumption is that preferences are separable in tobacco products. The assumption of separable preferences means that the decision-making process is tiered. With separability, an individual allocates his or her budget to broad categories: food, shelter, clothing, entertainment, and health. Then within each budget category, an independent and separate allocation of funds is made to various commodities in the budget category. Thus, within the food category, meat and vegetables are two possible subcategories. The meat subcategories might include chicken and beef. Finally, within the beef subcategory, there are two further categories: high-quality and low-quality beef.

Based on the consumer choice model (the one-goods[5] model in this study) in Deaton (1990), the demand function and the unit value function may be written as follows:

$$\ln v_{ic} = \alpha^1 + \beta^1 \ln x_{ic} + \psi \ln p_c + u_{ic}^1 \tag{2}$$

$$\ln q_{ic} = \alpha^0 + \varepsilon_x \ln x_{ic} + \varepsilon_p \ln p_c + \eta_c + u_{ic}^0 \tag{3}$$

where q_{ic} is the physical quantity of tobacco purchased by household i in cluster c, x_{ic} is the total expenditures of households i, p_c is the unobserved cluster price, η_c is the unobserved fixed cluster effect, v_{ic} is the unit value, and u_{ic} is the error term.

We assume that tobacco prices do not vary within clusters and are not observable. In Eq. (2), log unit value is regressed on log total expenditure and log actual prices with the exception of the cluster-fixed effect (this is a crucial assumption). In Eq. (3), the log quantity of the tobacco product is regressed on log total expenditure and log actual price by controlling the cluster-fixed effect. Note that we do not include the cluster-fixed effect on the right side of Eq. (2). Assume that the cluster effect is uncorrelated with actual market prices.

By substituting Eq. (2) into Eq. (3), we get

$$\ln q_{ic} = \alpha^0 - \frac{\varepsilon_x}{\psi}\alpha^1 + \varepsilon_x\left(1 - \frac{\beta^1}{\psi}\right)\ln x_{ic} + \frac{\varepsilon_p}{\psi}\ln v_{ic} + \eta_c + u_{ic}^0 - \frac{1}{\psi}u_{ic}^1 \tag{4}$$

The coefficient of unit value is $\frac{\varepsilon_p}{\psi}$, which is not price elasticity. Rather, it is the price elasticity of demand divided by the price elasticity of quality. The above equation could be estimated using OLS. Our aim is to estimate ε_p, the price elasticity of demand, rather than $\frac{\varepsilon_p}{\psi}$.

---

[5] In a multi-goods model, one can estimate both own-price elasticity and cross-price elasticity.

Modeling Quality

In the standard consumer model, expenditure equals price multiplied by quantity. If quality is introduced into the model, expenditure is the product of quality, quantity, and price. We assume that the marginal rate of substitution between different goods in the product group is independent of the quantities consumed outside the group. Then subgroup demand functions for the goods (such as tobacco) inside the group will always exist (Deaton & Muellbauer, 1980b). After some algebraic calculations (Deaton, 1997), the following equation is established:

$$\psi = 1 + \beta^1 \varepsilon_p / \varepsilon_x$$

We define $\phi = \frac{\varepsilon_p}{\psi}$. Combining the above two equations, we eventually arrive at price elasticity

$$\varepsilon_p = \frac{\phi}{1 - \phi\beta^1/\varepsilon_x} \tag{5}$$

Estimation Procedure

Deaton (1997) suggests a two-stage procedure for estimating price elasticity. In Eq. (5), we need estimates and $\phi = \frac{\varepsilon_p}{\psi}$, β^1, and ε_x.

First stage

As discussed in Sections 3.2 and 3.3, we can consistently estimate β^1 and ε_x in Eqs. (2) and (3) using the information within the clusters, that is, by including cluster dummies.

Second stage

This stage uses the information between clusters to estimate price elasticity. Once the first stage is complete, we can construct the following variables:

$$y_{ic}^0 = \ln q_{ic} - \hat{\varepsilon}_x \ln x_{ic}$$
$$y_{ic}^1 = \ln v_{ic} - \hat{\beta}_1 \ln x_{ic}$$

Then we calculated the following:

the cluster average of $y_c^0 = AVERAGE(y_{ic}^0)$, and

the cluster average of $y_c^1 = AVERAGE(y_{ic}^1)$

Deaton (1997) suggests that

$$\hat{\phi} \frac{\text{cov}(y^0 y^1) - \sigma^{01}/n_c}{\text{var}(y^1) - \sigma^{11}/n_c}$$

where σ^{01} and σ^{11} are the covariance of residuals from Eqs. (2) and (3) and the variance of the residual from Eq. (2). Finally, $\hat{\phi}, \hat{\beta}_1, \hat{\varepsilon}_x$ are substituted into Eq. (5) to obtain the actual price elasticity:

$$\hat{\varepsilon}_p = \frac{\hat{\phi}}{1 - \hat{\phi}\beta_1/\hat{\varepsilon}_x}$$

DATA AND DESCRIPTIVE STATISTICS

Data

UHIES, a population representative survey that covers about 25,000 urban households in China and is annually conducted by the National Bureau of Statistics (NBS),[6] uses a stratified design and probabilistic sampling. The survey provides data for a variety of household-level variables, including income, consumption, expenditures, demographics, and other household characteristics. UHIES is the only source of relevant information on household income, consumption, and expenditures for all kinds of goods in China. The data used in our study are a subsample of UHIES. The sample covers households in eight provinces[7] during 1999–2001.

UHIES data are used in this study for several reasons. According to some research (Chamon & Prasad, 2008; Ravallion & Chen, 1997), the quality of UHIES data is very high. Furthermore, this survey includes a large enough quantity of households to conduct empirical studies based on the resulting data. Perhaps the most important point is that this data set provides tobacco consumption and expenditure data at the household-level, which is necessary to estimate household responses to tobacco price.

---

[6]The sample size was about 25,000 in 1999–2001 and increased to 40,000 after 2001.

[7]One issue is whether our 8-province sample is a representative subset of the full UHIES sample. Chamon and Prasad (2008) have pointed out that no major discrepancies were found between the results using data for the subsample and results reported with data for the full sample for selected years.

We use stratification at the provincial level, that is, households are identified by province. In addition, because the consumption of leaf tobacco is so low, we analyze only cigarette consumption. The main variables utilized correspond to tobacco consumption, tobacco expenditure, household expenditure, location, disposable income, gender, education, employment of the head of household, and other individual characteristics. Household expenditures also are available on other daily necessities including food, potatoes, oil fats, eggs, aquatic product, vegetables, cigarettes, fruit, nuts, and cakes. The consumption quantity was aggregated over different qualities and varieties.

Table 1 summarizes the figures corresponding to the following demographic variables: income, consumption, and expenditures for the head of household and the entire household. We pooled the data for 1999, 2000, and 2001 into one data set (16,441 observations) in which about 72% of households included smokers. Some unreasonable values were eliminated from the observations. After data cleaning, the data set included 11,889 observations.

Table 1:   Variable Descriptions: 1999–2001

Variable Type	Variables	Mean	Std. Dev.	Min	Max
Head of household	Gender	1.20	0.40	1	2
	Age	43.09	8.42	21	75
	Education	3.63	1.41	1	7
	Industry	8.01	4.72	1	16
	Employment	1.64	1.45	1	7
	Vocation	43.21	23.41	11	80
	Total revenue	10,276.45	6,039.82	0	89,856
Household-level	Household size	3.12	0.66	1	7
(per capita	Disposable income	6,154.66	3,727.34	395	62,755
in one year,	Consumption expenditure	4,908.06	3,483.48	313	97,765
except household	Non-consumption	1,235.79	4,328.79	0	139,023
size variable)	expenditure				
	Food expenditure	1,800.32	972.86	43	11,559
	Cigarette consumption	30.63	43.98	0	545
	Cigarette expenditure	90.19	135.12	0	2,260
	Tobacco leaf consumption	0.03	0.28	0	11
	Tobacco leaf expenditure	0.33	2.86	0	94

Data source: The Urban Household Income and Expenditure Survey in China (1999–2001). The units of incomes and expenditures are nominal Yuan.

Descriptive Statistics

We are interested in the following issues: How many households have smokers? What is the quantity of tobacco consumption and expenditure in China? What is the price (unit value) of tobacco in China? Are there differences in tobacco consumption and unit value among income groups and regions? We also want to know what share of total household expenditures is represented by tobacco expenditures. Table 2 shows the results by average household. The most frequent response for leaf tobacco consumption was 0 in the cleaned sample (1.44% of the 11,889 households). This finding implies that most smokers in urban areas consumed just cigarettes and not leaf tobacco. Thus, in the following sections, we analyze only cigarette consumption. The share of households with smokers was between 70% and 75% consistently during this period. That is, most family members were directly or indirectly influenced by tobacco. In those households with smokers, cigarette consumption per capita per year was about 40 packs, cigarette expenditure per capita was 113–125 yuan, and tobacco expenditure as a share of food consumption was between 6.6% and 6.9% from 1999 to 2001. At the same time, unit value rose slightly from 2.80 to 3.04. The average unit value of the pooling data was 2.93 yuan/pack.

Table 2 shows the results at the provincial level. First, the share of households with smokers was between 60% and 80% in most provinces. Second, significant differences were found regarding cigarette expenditure in different provinces during this period; expenditure ranged between 30 yuan and 50 yuan. The cigarette expenditure in most provinces rose quite a bit from 1999 to 2001. One reason for this increase was that unit value increased. The disparity between the unit value figures for different provinces provides support for the assumption of regional price variation in the Deaton model.

In the next section, we examine cigarette consumption within different income groups. The households in the sample were divided into three groups according to disposable income per capita. We wished to know whether the wealthier households consumed more cigarettes. Table 3 shows that the share of households with smokers decreased from higher income tertiles to lower ones, both during each year and in the pooling data. In addition, cigarette consumption and expenditures did increase with income tertiles during the period. The unit value for the rich was also larger than that for the poor

Table 2:   Descriptive Statistics: Provincial Level (Household Average)

	Year	Total	Prov-1	Prov-2	Prov-3	Prov-4	Prov-5	Prov-6	Prov-7	Prov-8
Proportion	2001	70.84%	59.47%	78.93%	70.95%	74.37%	78.15%	68.58%	70.44%	68.83%
of households	2000	75.25%	65.92%	85.30%	75.85%	82.12%	78.75%	70.53%	68.01%	76.10%
with smokers	1999	72.49%	65.27%	78.15%	69.96%	76.08%	82.24%	70.14%	69.83%	70.96%
Cigarette	2001	41.16	50.22	49.61	45.35	38.02	31.50	50.42	32.76	35.38
consumption	2000	40.29	50.77	48.91	40.74	41.15	33.18	48.05	33.76	32.53
per capita	1999	40.69	46.32	54.91	39.41	44.00	30.84	47.24	33.30	34.07
Cigarette	2001	125.04	166.59	127.67	137.25	130.67	109.91	157.97	80.79	101.99
expenditure	2000	119.39	176.55	119.29	122.37	135.15	105.33	153.72	78.10	91.31
per capita	1999	113.88	158.9	134.99	104.56	144.84	92.68	130.73	75.32	88.45
Tobacco as	2001	6.64%	5.15%	4.86%	7.82%	9.88%	7.42%	7.59%	4.90%	6.34%
proportion of	2000	6.84%	5.54%	5.14%	7.32%	10.11%	7.80%	7.72%	5.12%	5.94%
food expenditure	1999	6.61%	5.16%	5.60%	6.21%	10.67%	7.24%	7.08%	5.05%	6.35%
Unit value	2001	3.04	3.32	2.57	3.03	3.44	3.49	3.13	2.47	2.88
	2000	2.96	3.48	2.44	3.00	3.28	3.17	3.20	2.31	2.81
	1999	2.80	3.43	2.46	2.65	3.29	3.01	2.77	2.26	2.60

Note: The units of cigarette consumption, cigarette expenditure, and unit value are pack, yuan, and yuan/pack, respectively. All the values in the table are calculated only by households with smokers, except "Proportion of households with smokers".

Table 3: Descriptive Statistics: By Income Groups (Household Average)

	Year	1st tertile	2nd tertile	3rd tertile
Proportion of households with smokers	Pooling	75.63%	72.89%	69.95%
	2001	73.36%	72.30%	66.87%
	2000	77.32%	75.63%	72.80%
	1999	77.14%	70.69%	69.64%
Cigarette consumption per capita	Pooling	35.19	39.07	49.30
	2001	35.15	41.47	48.31
	2000	34.40	37.47	50.58
	1999	35.83	37.57	50.09
Cigarette expenditure per capita	Pooling	81.32	116.32	169.36
	2001	88.82	125.63	169.54
	2000	78.43	113.69	175.41
	1999	78.64	108.37	163.67
Tobacco as proportion of food expenditure	Pooling	6.93%	6.62%	6.62%
	2001	7.19%	6.72%	6.26%
	2000	6.94%	6.53%	7.02%
	1999	6.75%	6.42%	6.66%
Unit value	Pooling	2.31	2.98	3.44
	2001	2.53	3.03	3.51
	2000	2.28	3.03	3.47
	1999	2.19	2.88	3.27

Note: The units of cigarette consumption, cigarette expenditure, and unit value are pack, yuan, and yuan/pack, respectively. All the values in the table are calculated only by households with smokers, except "Proportion of households with smokers". The pooling data are the 1999, 2000, and 2001 data combined.

each year. This finding means that high-income households consumed more cigarettes and faced higher unit values than did low-income households.

ECONOMETRIC TESTS

Two-part Model and Provincial Fixed Effect

First, we used the two-part model, which separates tobacco demand into smoking participation and smoking intensity (Lance *et al.*, 2004):

$$E(q) = Pr(q > 0) \times E(q|q > 0) \tag{6}$$

where q is household cigarette consumption. The elasticity of unconditional demand is

$$\eta_t = \eta_{\text{Pr}(q>0)} + \eta_{E(q|q>0)} \tag{7}$$

In the logit participation and log-linear intensity equations, the independent variables are log income, log mean price, age, education, gender, and other characteristics of the head of household.[8] The dependent variable in the logit model is a dichotomous variable equal to 1 for households with smokers and 0 for households without smokers.

The results are shown in Table 4. The participation elasticity is $-(1 - \text{Pr}(\text{Smoking} = 1)) \times 0.2976 = -0.0804$, which is a relatively small figure. The intensity elasticity is -0.7425, and the overall price elasticity is -0.8229. The small rate of participation elasticity also means that the estimation of the Deaton model that dropped the households without smokers and calculated the figure for intensity elasticity directly may be quite accurate.

Table 4: Two-part Model and Provincial Fixed Effect Model: Pooling Data

Model	Two-part Model		Provincial Fixed Effect Model
	Smoking Participation	Smoking Intensity	
Log income	0.1783***	0.5910***	0.6314***
	(0.0332)	(0.0238)	(0.0265)
Log price	−0.2976**	−0.7425***	−0.8146***
	(0.1389)	(0.0244)	(0.0249)
Household size	0.1132***	0.1025***	0.0895***
	(0.0229)	(0.0154)	(0.0154)
Intercept	−0.6405	−2.0188**	−2.3363***
	(1.2058)	(0.7879)	(0.8000)
Obs	16,439	11841	11841

Note: All the models are significant. *, **, *** denotes significance at the 10%, 5% and 1% levels, respectively. Standard errors are in the parentheses. The coefficients of demographic dummies, such as education, gender, and vocational are not listed in this table for simplicity.

---

[8]We also put the dummies of individual characteristics into the regression, and the results were very similar.

We also controlled for the provincial fixed effect in the following basic regression:

$$\ln q = \alpha + \varepsilon_x \ln x + \beta \ln p + \gamma PD + u \qquad (8)$$

where x is total household expenditure, p is tobacco price (unit value), PD is a vector of provincial dummies, and u is an error item. Thus, β is price elasticity and ε_x is income elasticity. The price elasticity of intensity is -0.8146, which is very close to the figure for overall elasticity achieved using the two-part model. This also indicates the small smoking participation elasticity of Chinese households.

The Deaton Model

The Deaton model assumes that the prices of commodities do not vary within each cluster. Because price is not included in the household survey, it is impossible to directly obtain parameter estimates for price directly. Nevertheless, we can consistently estimate the non-price parameters if we assume that all households in the same cluster are offered products with the same prices so that the local demand can be used to determine the quality elasticity. In such cases, the price variation across locations is used to measure price elasticity.

We first tested the assumption of regional variations in unit value. The log unit value was regressed on the cluster-fixed effects (that is, province dummies) by year. The results show strong evidence of inter-provincial price differences (in Table 5). F-tests tell us that all of these regressions are significant. If the three years are pooled into one data set, there will be $8 \times 3 = 24$ clusters (8 provinces $\times$ 3 years).[9] The results of the pooling cases also indicate the existence of regional price variation.

Next, we used the two-stage procedure associated with the Deaton model to estimate the price, quality, and income elasticity of tobacco consumption for Chinese households. In the first stage, within-cluster information on household demand, income, and unit value was used to obtain estimates of the quality effect. Demographic dummies for the head of household, such as

---

[9]The province in different years is viewed as another cluster. We assumed cigarette prices do not vary within each year and do not vary within each geographic location, so the change in prices between years is similar across clusters.

Table 5:   Unit Value on Provincial Fixed Effects: 1999–2001

Log Unit Value	2001	2000	1999
Pdm(1)	0.3102***	(Dropped)	0.2676***
	(0.0447)		(0.0460)
Pdm(2)	(Dropped)	−0.2576***	(Dropped)
		(0.0525)	
Pdm(3)	0.1402*	−0.1126**	0.0821**
	(0.0415)	(0.0510)	(0.0412)
Pdm(4)	0.2755***	−0.0466	0.2015***
	(0.0399)	(0.0503)	(0.0407)
Pdm(5)	0.3068***	0.0134	0.1346*
	(0.0406)	(0.0520)	(0.0416)
Pdm(6)	0.2256***	0.0207	0.0391***
	(0.0372)	(0.0488)	(0.0386)
Pdm(7)	−0.0305	−0.2996***	−0.1427*
	(0.0396)	(0.0514)	(0.0413)
Pdm(8)	0.0843**	−0.1367*	0.0008
	(0.0378)	(0.0486)	(0.0390)
Intercept	0.9540***	1.1807***	0.9803***
	(0.0302)	(0.0429)	(0.0310)

Note: *, **, *** denotes significance at the 10%, 5% and 1% levels, respectively. Standard errors are in the parentheses. Pdm(n) is the nth provincial dummy.

age and age squared, also were controlled for in regression Eqs. (2) and (3). Then cluster means were subtracted from the independent variables in Eqs. (2) and (3). These equations were estimated using OLS to obtain ε_x and $\hat{\beta}^1$.

Table 6 shows the income, quality, and price elasticity of cigarette consumption for all households estimated via the Deaton methodology both year-by-year and using pooling data. The income elasticity ranged from 0.27 to 0.45 during 1999 and 2001. In other words, if the income of a household increases by 1%, the quantity of cigarettes consumed will increase by 0.27% to 0.45%. Quality elasticity refers to changes in the quality of the products purchased as they correspond to changes in household income. The quality elasticity was about 0.3 in this case. All of the price elasticity figures were negative, and there were obvious differences during the period. In 1999, the price elasticity was −0.4788. That figure declined to −0.5603 in 2000, and then in 2001, it rose to −0.3526 instead. If we use the pooling data rather than each year's data independently to estimate the model, the price elasticity

Table 6: Price Elasticity, Quality Elasticity, and Income Elasticity

	Year	Total	1st tertile	2nd tertile	3rd tertile
Price elasticity	Pooling	−0.4325	−0.4554	−0.4224	−0.4176
	2001	−0.3526	−0.3696	−0.3797	−0.3249
	2000	−0.5603	−0.6967	−0.6133	−0.5065
	1999	−0.4788	−0.7003	−0.5674	−0.4272
Quality elasticity	Pooling	0.3160	0.2781	0.1946	0.3352
	2001	0.3158	0.3426	0.1316	0.2291
	2000	0.3366	0.2613	0.3049	0.3937
	1999	0.3000	0.2376	0.1799	0.3021
Income elasticity	Pooling	0.3621	0.5021	0.3389	0.3519
	2001	0.2747	0.3642	0.2553	0.3369
	2000	0.4489	0.4755	0.3513	0.5693
	1999	0.3528	0.7001	0.2207	0.2925
Obs.	Pooling	8658	2994	2891	2773

Note: In all the models, two regressions (2) and (3) in the first stage are significant. The observations from the pooling data regressions are listed in the last line.

becomes −0.4325. We also estimated income, quality, and price elasticities by income groups because different income groups might exhibit different patterns of tobacco demand. We found that in most cases, a pattern emerged in which the 1st tertile group was most responsive to increased price (or tax). However, a few outliers were not consistent with this pattern, possibly reflecting the small samples on which the estimates were based. Thus, changes in tobacco control policy, especially excise taxes, will have different effects on households with different income levels. However, from the results in Table 6, we cannot conclude that the low-income group had lower income elasticity and the high-income group had higher income elasticity. In every period from 1999 to 2001, the second tertile group had the smallest income elasticity. When the data were pooled, the same results emerged.

Our finding of relatively high price elasticity of cigarette consumption is consistent with results presented by Nicita (2004) and John (2005), who also used the Deaton method. Nicita (2004) estimated a demand system that includes 11 goods. His results showed that the price elasticity of alcohol and tobacco (combined into one good) was −0.91 in Mexico during the period from 1989 to 2000. John (2005) calculated the own-price elasticities of six types of tobacco in India. Their elasticities ranged between −0.6 and −1.0.

Sensitivity Tests: Demand System Analysis

In this section, we estimate two demand systems of households to run sensitivity tests. Ten products are included in our demand systems: food, potatoes, oil fats, eggs, aquatic product, vegetables, cigarettes, fruit, nuts, and cakes. These products are indexed by i, i = 1 . . . 10. Based on the method of Stone's Analysis, the system is as follows:

$$\ln q_i = \alpha_i + e_i \left\{ \ln X - \sum_k \omega_k \ln p_k \right\} + \sum_{k=1}^{n} e_{ik}^* \ln p_k + \varepsilon_i \qquad (9)$$

where q_i is the consumption of commodity i, p_i is the unit value of commodity i, X is the total consumption expense, and ω_i is the budget share of commodity i. The own- and cross-price elasticities for these 10 products can be obtained by regressing these equations. The own-price elasticity of cigarettes was -0.5731. If the households are divided into three groups, we find that the own-price elasticity of cigarettes for the 1st tertile group is -0.6736 and -0.5253 for the 2nd tertile group and -0.5285 for the 3rd tertile group.

The second method used here is that of flexible functional forms (Deaton, 1986; Pollak & Wales, 1992). We use only one type of the flexible functional forms: AIDS (Deaton & Muellbauer, 1980a). We defined the commodity's budget share as the expenditure on this commodity divided by the total expenditure on all commodities included in the demand system. w_i represents the budget share of commodity i. The regressions are specified as follows:

$$w_i = \alpha_i + \beta_i \ln (X/P) + \sum_{j=1}^{N} \gamma_{ij} \ln p_j + \varepsilon_i \qquad (10)$$

where w_i represents the budget share of commodity i. P is an overall price index for the commodities, p_j is the price of the jth commodity, and j = 1 . . . 10. The log price index (log P) can have a different form. It is common to employ a linear approximation, which allows for a more straightforward estimation of the model parameters (i.e., LA/AIDS). In particular, Deaton and Muellbauer (1980a) have suggested the "Stone Price Index," defined as follows:

$$\ln P = \sum_{i=1}^{N} w_i \ln p_i.$$

The index is a weighted average of commodity prices, with commodities' average budget shares (w_i) as weights. The constraints of the demand system (Eq. (10)) are as follows: *Adding up*, $\Sigma_i \alpha_i = 1$, $\Sigma_i \beta_i = 0$; *Homogeneity*, $\Sigma_j \gamma_{ij} = 0$; and *Symmetry*, $\gamma_{ij} = \gamma_{ji}$. Because the dependent variable is budget share, the error covariance matrix is singular. Thus, we must drop one equation from the demand system (Eq. (10)), the last one (the cake regression). Zellner's seemingly unrelated regression (SUR) technique is used to estimate this demand system. Chalfant (1987) has suggested that under LA/AIDS, the own-price elasticity is as follows:

$$\eta_{ii} = \frac{\gamma_{ii}}{w_i} \beta_i - 1$$

Cross-price elasticity is:

$$\eta_{ij} = \frac{\gamma_{ii}}{w_i} \beta_i \left(\frac{w_j}{w_i} \right)$$

Expenditure elasticity is:

$$\eta_i = \frac{\beta_i}{w_i} + 1.$$

As shown in Table 7, the price elasticity of cigarette demand was -0.8125, and the corresponding expenditure elasticity was 1.4173. These are very high figures.

TAX POLICY ON TOBACCO CONSUMPTION: MICRO-SIMULATION

Policymakers view a tobacco tax as a disincentive to tobacco consumption in many countries. In this section, we use a simple simulation to analyze the impact of tobacco tax policy on tobacco consumption and fiscal revenue using the price elasticities estimated in the previous section.

In 2005, the average consumption of cigarettes in China was 72 packs per capita, and national consumption was 94.1 billion packs. The average retail price of a pack of 20 cigarettes was 4.52 yuan (which equals 0.65 dollar). Currently, China has two excise taxes on cigarettes: a specific tax and an ad valorem tax. The specific excise is 0.06 yuan per pack. The ad valorem tax is 30% of the producer price if the producer price is less than 5 yuan per pack;

Table 7:   Price and Expenditure Elasticities in Demand
Systems: Pooling Data

	Price Elasticity	Income Elasticity
Food	−1.0994	0.9878
Potatoes	−1.0726	1.0535
Oil	−0.5369	0.8846
Eggs	−0.8848	0.8399
Aquatic Product	−0.1283	0.9387
Vegetable	−0.7483	1.0808
Cigarettes	−0.8125	1.4173
Fruit	−0.6867	0.9222
Nuts	−0.2922	0.8272
Cakes	−0.2170	0.3716

Note: Ten products are included in the AIDS demand
system: food, potatoes, oil fats, eggs, aquatic product,
vegetable, cigarettes, fruit, nuts, and cakes. Zellner's
seemingly unrelated regression (SUR) technique is used
to estimate this AIDS demand system.

otherwise, it is 45%.[10] According to Sunley (2008), the total tobacco tax in
China was only 32% of the retail price in 2005. Hu *et al.* (2008) cite a figure of
40% when the tax on one pack is 1.81 yuan. This is a relatively low percentage
compared with tobacco taxes in other countries (which tend to be 65%–70%
on average).

Our simulation requires two assumptions: (1) no substitution effect due to
price increases and (2) price elasticity does not change from year to year so the
tax is the only factor influencing price. Assuming that cigarette consumption
in China is 94.1 billion packs per year, that the price of cigarettes is 4.52 yuan
per pack, and that the total tobacco tax per pack is 40%, then the fiscal revenue
from cigarette excise taxes in one year equals 94.1*4.52*40% = 170.13 billion
yuan.

A great deal of research has suggested that governments should adjust
their specific tobacco taxes. Our policy simulations use tax increases of 0.5,
1.0, 1.5, 2.0, 2.5, 3.0, 3.5, and 4.0 yuan per pack (the initial price is 5.02
yuan). In Table 8, the first row displays the simulation results that correspond

---

[10]In addition, cigarettes in China are also subject to the 17% VAT.

Table 8: Simulations with Estimated Parameters

	Δt	0.50	1.00	1.50	2.00	2.50	3.00	3.50	4.00
	Price	5.02	5.52	6.02	6.52	7.02	7.52	8.02	8.52
Price Elasticity	Δ Price	11.06%	22.12%	33.19%	44.25%	55.31%	66.37%	77.43%	88.50%
Consumption	−0.3526	−3.67	−7.34	−11.01	−14.68	−18.35	−22.02	−25.69	−29.36
Increasing	−0.4325	−4.50	−9.00	−13.51	−18.01	−22.51	−27.01	−31.52	−36.02
(Billion Packs)	−0.4788	−4.98	−9.97	−14.95	−19.94	−24.92	−29.90	−34.89	−39.87
	−0.5603	−5.83	−11.66	−17.50	−23.33	−29.16	−34.99	−40.82	−46.66
	−0.5731	−5.97	−11.93	−17.90	−23.86	−29.83	−35.79	−41.76	−47.73
	−0.8044	−8.37	−16.75	−25.12	−33.49	−41.87	−50.24	−58.61	−66.99
	−0.8125	−8.46	−16.92	−25.37	−33.83	−42.29	−50.75	−59.21	−67.66
Government	−0.3526	38.57	73.48	104.71	132.27	156.16	176.39	192.94	205.82
Revenue	−0.4325	36.65	68.80	96.44	119.58	138.22	152.36	161.99	167.13
Increasing	−0.4788	35.54	66.09	91.66	112.24	127.84	138.46	144.09	144.74
(Billion Yuan)	−0.5603	33.58	61.32	83.24	99.32	109.57	113.99	112.58	105.33
	−0.5731	33.27	60.57	81.91	97.28	106.69	110.13	107.61	99.12
	−0.8044	27.71	47.04	58.00	60.59	54.81	40.65	18.12	−12.79
	−0.8125	27.51	46.57	57.16	59.30	52.98	38.20	14.97	−16.73

Note: Assuming cigarette consumption in China is 94.1 billion packs per year, the price of cigarettes is 4.52 yuan per pack, and the total tobacco tax per pack is 40%. Policy simulations use tax increases of 0.5,1.0,1.5, 2.0, 2.5, 3.0, 3.5, and 4.0 yuan per pack respectively.

to various tax increases. The second row is the new price after a particular tax increase. The third row is the percentage change in the price of one pack. Then we let price elasticities equal the elasticities estimated in the earlier sections. We find that cigarette consumption decreases rapidly and fiscal revenue increases rapidly as the tax increases. However, if the excise tax increases too much, the government revenue from the tobacco excise tax will decrease. Based on different price elasticities, policymakers in China could legitimately raise the tax burden on tobacco consumption, which might both increase fiscal revenue and curb tobacco consumption.

In the simulation, the elasticities included the two-part model, the Deaton model estimations, and the demand system estimations. If the price elasticity is −0.4325, as is estimated based on pooling the data, then cigarette consumption will drop by 4.50 billion packs per year, and the government will obtain more than 36.65 billion yuan when the tobacco tax increases 0.5 yuan. If the elasticity is −0.8125, then cigarette consumption will drop by 8.46 billion packs and the government will obtain more than 27.51 billion yuan in revenue.

CONCLUSION

Tobacco taxes have been proven as an effective tool for controlling tobacco consumption. Because taxation is basically a method of raising tobacco prices, one must know the price elasticity of tobacco demand to test the impact of a particular tax hike on tobacco consumption. This study has used a new data set and several complicated demand models to develop new evidence of the behavior parameters of Chinese households. We also simulated excise tax policies to test their impact on tobacco consumption and the potential fiscal revenue from various increases.

Based on the two-part model and provincial fixed-effects model, the overall price elasticity is about -0.82. The Deaton models showed that when we considered the quality effect, the price elasticity of cigarettes was between -0.70 and -0.35. That is, if the price of cigarettes increases, consumers will reduce their cigarette consumption even if they can choose to consume a lower quality of cigarette with a similar expenditure on tobacco products. These are relatively high price elasticities. Furthermore, the price elasticities estimated using Stone's method and the AIDS model were -0.57 and -0.81, respectively.

Our study has several limitations that should be acknowledged. First, this study estimated the demand elasticity of households only. Tobacco price elasticity at the individual level also needs to be estimated via survey. Second, we used a sample of urban households in eight provinces in North China, so the estimations may reflect specific regional price elasticity figures for tobacco. A national survey including urban and rural areas should be used to analyze tobacco consumption. Finally, while we tackled the endogeneity issue by employing the Deaton method, another important problem that we encountered in these household surveys is measurement error. This problem needs to be addressed in the future. More precise and in-depth research on China's tobacco consumption and welfare analysis must be conducted if we are to make additional progress toward tobacco control in China.

ACKNOWLEDGMENTS

This study is part of the Tobacco Economics and Taxation Project supported by the World Health Organization (WHO), Bloomberg Foundation and Johns Hopkins University. We also acknowledges the support by the Humanities and Social Science Fund of MOE (10YJC790077), and the National Science Foundation of China (No. 71073002 and 70903003). We are grateful to Ayda Yurekli, Teh-wei Hu, Frank Chaloupka, Richard Peck, Hugh Waters, Petit Patrick, Stephen Tamplin, Gauri Khanna, Sarah England, Xin Xu, Zhiyong Yang, Xiaoyun Zhang, Rose Zheng, Huan Liu, Gongliang Tang, Xiangyi Meng, and Song Gao for helpful comments. All errors are our own.

REFERENCES

Baltagi, B., Griffin, J., & Xiong, W. (2000). To pool or not to pool: Homogeneous versus heterogeneous estimators applied to cigarette demand. *The Review of Economics and Statistics*, 82(1), 117–126.

Becker, G. S., & Murphy, K. M. (1988). A theory of rational addiction. *Journal of Political Economy*, 96(4), 675–700.

Bishop, J., Liu, H., & Meng, Q. (2007). Are Chinese smokers sensitive to price? *China Economic Review*, 18, 113–121.

Chalfant, J. A. (1987). A globally flexible, almost ideal demand system. *Journal of Business and Economic Statistics*, 5(2), 233–242.

Chaloupka, F. J., & Warner, K. E. (2000). The economics of smoking. In A. J. Culyer, & J. P. Newhouse (Eds.), *Handbook of health economics, vol. 1.* (pp. 1539–1627) Amsterdam: North-Holland.

Chamon, M., & Prasad, E., 2008. *Why are Saving Rates of Urban Households in China Rising?* NBER Working Paper No. 14546.

Chapman, S., & Richardson, J. (1990). Tobacco excise and declining tobacco consumption: The case of Papua New Guinea. *American Journal of Public Health*, 80(5), 537–540.

Cragg, J. G. (1971). Some statistical models for limited dependent variables with application to the demand for durable goods. *Econometrica*, 39(5), 829–844.

Crawford, I., Laisney, F., & Preston, I. (2003). Estimation of household demand systems with theoretically compatible engel curves and unit value specification. *Journal of Econometrics*, 114, 221–241.

Deaton, A. (1986). Demand analysis. In Z. Griliches, & M. Intriligator (Eds.), *Handbook of econometrics, vol. 3.* (pp. 1767–1839) Amsterdam: North-Holland.

Deaton, A. (1988). Quality, quantity, and spatial variation of price. *The American Economic Review*, 78(3), 418–430.

Deaton, A. (1989). Household survey data and pricing policies in developing countries. *World Bank Economic Review*, 3(2), 183–210.

Deaton, A. (1990). Price elasticities from survey data: Extensions and Indonesian results. *Journal of Econometrics*, 44, 281–309.

Deaton, A. (1997). *The analysis of household surveys: A microeconometric approach to development policy.* Baltimore and London: The Johns Hopkins University Press.

Deaton, A., & Muellbauer, J. (1980a). An almost ideal demand system. *The American Economic Review*, 70(3), 312–326.

Deaton, A., & Muellbauer, J. (1980b). *Economics and consumer behavior.* New York: Cambridge University Press.

Escario, J., & Molina, J. A. (2004). Modeling the optimal fiscal policy on tobacco consumption. *Journal of Policy Modeling,* 26, 81–93.

Hu, T. W., Mao, Z., Shi, J., & Chen, W. (2008). *Tobacco taxation and its potential impact in China.* Paris: International Union against Tuberculosis and Lung Disease.

John, R.M., 2005. *Price elasticity estimates for tobacco and other addictive goods in India.* Working Papers 2005-003, Indira Gandhi Institute of Development Research, Mumbai, India.

Lance, P., Akin, J., Dow, W., & Loh, C. (2004). Is cigarette smoking in poorer nations highly sensitive to price? Evidence from Russia and China. *Journal of Health Economics,* 23, 173–189.

Mao, Z., & Hu, D. (2008). Research on cigarette demand and the influencing factors (in Chinese). In D. Hu, & Z. Mao (Eds.), *Economics researches on tobacco control in China.* Beijing: Economic Science Press.

Mao, Z., Hu, D., & Yang, G. (2005). New evaluating of the demand for cigarettes from Chinese residents (in Chinese). *Chinese Health Economics,* 25(5), 45–47.

Mao, Z., Yang, G., Ma, J., Samet, J., & Ceraso, M. (2003). Adults' demand for cigarettes and its influencing factors in China (in Chinese). *Soft Science of Health,* 17(2), 19–22.

Nicita, A., 2004. *Efficiency and Equity of a Marginal Tax Reform — Income, Quality, and Price Elasticities for Mexico.* Policy Research Working Paper Series 3266, The World Bank.

Niimi, Y., 2005. *An Analysis of Household Responses to Price Shocks in Vietnam: Can Unit Values Substitute for Market Prices?* PRUS Working Paper, No. 30, Poverty Research Unit at Sussex, University of Sussex.

Pogue, T., & Sgontz, L. (1989). Taxing to control social costs: The case of alcohol. *The American Economic Review,* 79(1), 235–243.

Pollak, R., & Wales, T. (1992). *Demand system specification and estimation.* Oxford: Oxford University Press.

Prais, S. J., & Houthakker, H. S. (1955). *The analysis of family budgets.* Cambridge: Cambridge University Press.

Ravallion, M., & Chen, S. (1997). What can new survey data tell us about recent changes in distribution and poverty? *World Bank Economic Review,* 11(2), 357–382.

Sayginsoy, Y., & De Beyer, J. (2002). Cigarette demand, taxation, and the poor. *World Bank, Economics of Tobacco Control Paper, No. 4.*

Smith, Walter (2010). Who really benefits from cigarette tax? http://www.hvpress.net/news/119/ARTICLE/9021/2010-04-21.html.

Sunley, E. (2008). China: excises on cigarettes — A Way Forward, memo.

Sung, H. Y., Wang, L., Jin, S., Hu, T. W., & Jiang, Y. (2006). Economic burden of smoking in China, 2000. *Tobacco Control,* 15(Suppl 1), i5–i11.

Tansel, A. (1993). Cigarette demand, health scares and education in Turkey. *Applied Economics,* 25(4), 521–529.

Wilkins, N., Yurekli, A., & Hu, T. (2007). Economic analysis of tobacco demand. *World Bank, Economics of Tobacco Toolkit. Tool, 3.*

World Bank, Economics of tobacco toolkit (t). http://www1.worldbank.org/tobacco/toolkit.asp.

Yen, Steven T., Fang, Cheng, & Shew-Jiuan, Su. (2004). Household food demand in urban China: A censored system approach. *Journal of Comparative Economics*, 32(3), 564–585.

Young, G. H., Ma, J. M., Liu, N., & Zhou, L. N. (2005). Smoking and passive smoking in Chinese, (in Chinese). *Zhonghua Liu Xing Bing Xue Za Zhi*, 26(2), 77–83.

The Effect of Cigarette Prices on Brand-Switching in China: A Longitudinal Analysis of Data from the ITC China Survey*

Justin S. White, Jing Li, Teh-wei Hu, Geoffrey T. Fong and Yuan Jiang

ABSTRACT

Background Recent studies have found that Chinese smokers are relatively unresponsive to cigarette prices. As the Chinese government contemplates higher tobacco taxes, it is important to understand the reasons for this low response. One possible explanation is that smokers buffer themselves from rising cigarette prices by switching to cheaper cigarette brands.

Objective This study examines how cigarette prices influence consumers' choices of cigarette brands in China.

Methods This study uses panel data from the first three waves of the International Tobacco Control China Survey, drawn from six large cities in China and collected between 2006 and 2009. The study sample includes 3477 smokers who are present in at least two waves (8552 person-years). Cigarette brands are sorted by price into four tiers, using excise tax categories to determine the cut-off for each tier. The analysis

*Published in *Tob Control*, 2013; 00:1–7. doi: 10.1136/tobaccocontrol-2012-050922 (May 22, 2013).

relies on a conditional logit model to identify the relationship between price and brand choice.

Findings Overall, 38% of smokers switched price tiers from one wave to the next. A ¥1 change in the price of cigarettes alters the tier choice of 4–7% of smokers. Restricting the sample to those who chose each given tier at baseline, a ¥1 increase in price in a given tier would decrease the share choosing that tier by 4% for Tier 1 and 1–2% for Tiers 2 and 3.

Conclusions China's large price spread across cigarette brands appears to alter the brand selection of some consumers, especially smokers of cheaper brands. Tobacco pricing and tax policy can influence consumers' incentives to switch brands. In particular, whereas ad valorem taxes in a tiered pricing system like China's encourage trading down, specific excise taxes discourage the practice.

INTRODUCTION

Cigarettes are relatively affordable in China, and their affordability has increased with rising incomes over the last two decades.[1] Retail data from 2009 (described below) indicate that cigarettes are available in some urban areas for less than ¥2 per pack (approximately US$ 0.30). Such low-price cigarettes have been identified as a central impediment to smoking cessation.[2,3] A second feature of the cigarette market in China is the considerable variability of prices across brands. The range in prices per pack in Chinese stores routinely vary 10-fold and in some stores 50-fold or more. This wide price spread across brands makes it easy for smokers to switch to cheaper cigarettes in China, relative to other countries where the variability of prices is lower.

In the present study, we sought to understand the extent to which cigarette prices alter the purchasing decisions of smokers in China. The answer has profound health and policy implications for China's 300 million smokers.

Research over several decades has established that smokers are sensitive to changes in cigarette prices (e.g., Chaloupka and Warner).[4] The consensus estimate is that, on average — albeit with variation across studies, contexts, empirical specifications and estimation approaches typically falling between −0.2 and −0.6 — a 10% price increase is associated with a 4% decline in cigarette consumption, implying a price elasticity of −0.4.[5,6] (See the 2011 International Agency for Research on Cancer report and references therein for more discussion.[5]) Yet in China, the price elasticity of demand has been considerably lower, based on analyses of high-quality, individual-level data, although some older studies and time series analyses have found tobacco use in China to be more price-elastic.[7] Lance *et al.*[8] find a best estimate of −0.007 in nine Chinese provinces from 1993 to 1997. In an updated analysis, White and Hu[9] find similar price insensitivity over the subsequent decade. Mao *et al.*[10] use national data to estimate a price elasticity estimate of −0.15.[10] Huang *et al.*[11] estimate a price elasticity of consumption (i.e., excluding quit behaviour) of −0.13 between 2006 and 2009, using International Tobacco Control (ITC) Survey data. The overall lack of price sensitivity in China raises the public health concern that tobacco tax policy will have little impact on smoking behaviour.

Three potentially overlapping explanations may account for the low observed price elasticity in China. First, prices have changed little over time, and researchers lack sufficient price variation to identify the effect of prices on cigarette demand. Second, rising incomes have outpaced changes in cigarette prices, making cigarettes increasingly affordable over time and making it appear as though smokers do not respond to price changes. Third, the large spread in prices across cigarette brands enables Chinese smokers to buffer themselves against rising cigarette prices by switching to cheaper cigarette brands. Li *et al.* (2011) provide some empirical support for this latter hypothesis by showing that Chinese smokers who buy less-expensive brands tend to be less likely to intend to quit.[2] In addition, some studies have documented in other contexts an association between cigarette price and type of cigarette smoked.[12–17] Our study provides the first direct test of how price affects smokers' choice of cigarette brands in China. We do so in an empirical framework that also addresses the price variation hypothesis and controls for longitudinal changes in income. Our results highlight how pricing and tax policy in China alter consumers' incentives for choosing one brand over another.

METHODS

Data

Our data come from the ITC China Survey, a longitudinal survey of smoking behaviour among adults in China. We use the first three panels of the survey data, collected in 2006, 2007–2008 and 2009 in six capital cities: Beijing, Shanghai, Guangzhou, Shenyang, Changsha and Yinchuan. The ITC China Survey employs a multistage cluster sampling method to obtain a representative sample of adult smokers and non-smokers at the city level. In addition, individual-level sampling weights were constructed to estimate population characteristics. A more detailed description of the methodology of the ITC China Survey is presented in Wu et al.[18]

For the purpose of tracking the same individuals' brand choices at multiple points in time, we restricted the sample to the 4632 continuing smokers who participated in the ITC China Survey for at least two waves. After dropping those smokers for whom the tier choice could not reliably be determined, as discussed below, the final analytical sample included 3477 persons who constituted 8552 person-years (i.e., 8552 total observations in the analysis, roughly 2.5 per person). Overall retention in our selected sample is 82.0% which is relatively high.

Variables

Dependent variable

The dependent variable was a smoker's choice of cigarette price tier in each wave. Since this information was not readily available in the survey data, we constructed the dependent variable using the brand and price information of cigarettes last purchased by each smoker at the time of survey. Smokers were asked in each wave to provide the brand family, brand variety, total spending and quantity purchased when they last bought cigarettes for themselves, from which we determined the brand and per-pack price of cigarettes. The quantity last purchased is either the number of packs or the number of cartons (equal to 20 packs). Our analysis converts all prices into a per-pack equivalent.

We first validated the price data from the survey against cigarette retail price data collected in the six ITC cities at the same time that Wave 3 was fielded. The retail prices were very similar to average brand-specific prices in the Wave 3 survey data. We compared the city-level median price of the eight most commonly selected brand varieties in the survey data to those varieties' reported retail prices by city, and they were identical for five varieties and differed by less than ¥0.5 for the other three varieties. Next, we assigned to each observation a brand variety code using the ITC Project's classification scheme, based on the Universal Product Code on the barcode of each pack. For cases in which the interviewer entered a name in the 'Other' variety field, we manually assigned a brand variety code based on the names provided by respondents. Through these two routes, we were able to assign a brand variety code to 78%

Table 1: Cigarette Retail Prices in China by Tier, 2009

Tier	Retail Price (¥/pack)	Producer Profit (%)	Retail Profit (%)	Smokers (N)	Smokers (%)
1	[0, 2.65)	17.6	10.0	1114	13.2
2	[2.65, 5.15)	25.0	10.0	3830	45.3
3	[5.15, 8.97)	33.3	10.0	2345	27.7
4	[8.97, 18.95)	33.3	15.0	955	11.3
5	[18.95, 29.76)	40.8	15.0	150	1.8
6	[29.76, ∞)	51.5	15.0	59	0.7
				8453	100.0

Retail price ranges are calculated according to the formula (Gao, Zheng and Hu, 2011): Retail Price = Allocation Price × (1+Producer π) × (1+Retail π) × (1 + VAT), where π denotes profit and VAT is the value-added tax. The ranges for profits come from Gao, Zheng and Hu (2012). For retail price ranges, a bracket denotes a closed interval, and a parenthesis denotes an open interval. Tiers 4–6 are combined for analysis due to small cell sizes. Cell counts and proportions are survey weighted. The unweighted sample size is 8552 person-years from 3477 smokers.

of all observations involving continuing smokers, which constitutes our final sample. We calculated the median price for each brand variety in each city as the basis for assigning price tiers.

In order to sort brand varieties into price tiers, it is important to use a meaningful, exogenous source of information to determine the cut-off for each tier. We used the six-grade classification of cigarette allocation prices to calculate the retail price range for each grade, which is presented in Table 1. In China, allocation prices are similar to producer prices and serve as the basis for cigarette excise taxes. The allocation prices are drawn from China's State Tobacco Monopoly Administration, as reported in Gao, Zheng and Hu (2012).[19] We combined the three most expensive grades into one tier in our analysis because each of those tiers had very few observations. Hence our final classification of cigarette price has four tiers. We assigned a price tier to each observation based on the range into which its by-city median brand variety price falls.

Independent variables

The independent variable of interest is the nominal price of all tiers from which each smoker chooses. Our analyses depend on relative tier prices; thus, using real prices would have no impact on the analyses. For each tier, we use the median price of all corresponding brand varieties in each city at each wave. Our price measure thus represents the tier-specific market price smokers face in a given city and at a given wave. This measure should be insensitive to any non-systematic bias in smokers' self-reported price.

In addition, we control for a variety of demographic characteristics of smokers: gender, age, income at each wave, education at baseline and average number of cigarettes smoked per day at baseline. Gender, income and education information are coded as categorical variables and enter our model as dummy variables, whereas age and baseline quantity smoked are continuous variables. We also include tier-specific constants and control for the city and wave of each observation. As such, only those factors that vary temporally *and* geographically may bias our results. We have no evidence that omitted variables such as brand-specific advertising and marketing vary systematically by wave *and* by city.

Statistical Model

We employ a conditional logit framework,[20] which models the probability of a smoker choosing a given tier of cigarettes as a logit function of a linear combination of all independent

variables:

$$\Pr(Y_{it} = k) = \frac{\exp(V_{ikt})}{\sum_{j=1}^{4} \exp(V_{ikt})}, \quad k = 1, 2, 3, 4 \tag{1}$$

where

$$V_{ijt} = \alpha P_{ijt} + X_{ijt}\beta_j \tag{2}$$

In a given wave t, each smoker i chooses a price tier k from a menu of j tiers. Smoker i's cigarette tier choice is a logit function of the tier-specific price P_{ijt} and a vector of control variables X_{ijt}, described above. The coefficient of interest is α on tier price.

The conditional logit model differs from a standard logit model in that it allows for inclusion of alternative-specific variables, in this case cigarette prices that vary by tier. The regression includes four different price measures for each smoker, one for each tier, allowing us to take into account the full set of prices each smoker faced in his or her city at a given point in time. In addition to the regression coefficients, the analyses also allows us to estimate the average marginal effects of cigarette tier prices, that is, the change of probability in choosing a given cigarette tier resulting from a ¥1 increase in the median price of that tier. We computed the net marginal effects, accounting for movement in and out of a given tier, and the gross marginal effects, accounting only for movement out of a given tier. The net effects were calculated from the full sample, whereas the gross effects were calculated separately for each tier by restricting the sample to those smokers who used a given tier at baseline (i.e., in the earliest wave in which the smoker appeared in the sample). We computed bootstrapped standard errors for the average marginal effects, using 1000 repetitions and clustering at the individual level.

RESULTS

Descriptive Statistics

Table 1 shows the retail price ranges associated with each cigarette tier. About 45% of smokers chose a brand that falls in the second-cheapest tier (roughly ¥3–¥5 per pack). The next most commonly selected is the third-cheapest tier (28%, ¥5–¥9), followed by the cheapest tier (13%, ¥1–¥3). Only 2.5% of smokers last bought a pack in one of the two most expensive tiers, in which cigarettes cost more than ¥19. Retail prices are derived from government-regulated profit rates for producers and retailers. Allowable profit rates vary by tier, such that more expensive packs yield greater returns.

Figure 1 shows the degree to which smokers switch cigarette tiers across waves. A majority of smokers, between 50% and 71% depending on the tier and waves under consideration, stayed within the same price tier from wave to wave, yet a sizeable fraction switch cigarette tiers over time. Overall, 38% of smokers switched tiers from one survey round to the next. For mid-priced tiers (Tiers 2 and 3), in which a smoker could choose a more or less expensive brand, trading up to a more expensive tier tended to be more common than trading down. An exception is Tier 3 users in Wave 2, who were more likely to trade down in Wave 3. The general pattern of trading up may reflect that incomes rose faster than cigarette prices during this time period, providing cigarette users with additional purchasing power. Whereas tobacco prices increased a mere 1.5% nationally from 2006 to 2009, according to the official statistics

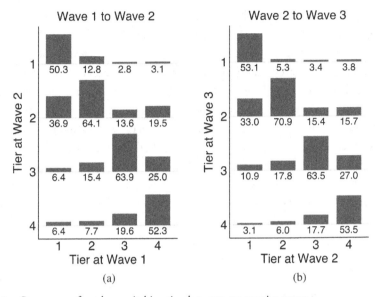

Fig 1:   Percentage of smokers switching tiers between consecutive waves.
Note: Column percentages are shown. (A) Displays switching from Wave 1 to Wave 2 among 2474 smokers. (B) Displays switching from Wave 2 to Wave 3 among 2240 smokers.

from the tobacco consumer price index,[21] average nominal incomes for urban residents rose 46% during this time period.[22]

According to the descriptive statistics presented in Table 2, more than 96% of the sample is men. The average age of smokers is 51 years. The average price of cigarettes purchased is ¥6.32 and the median price (not shown) is ¥5.00. Average nominal and real cigarette prices in 2006 terms are nearly identical, due to very low growth in the consumer price index for tobacco products during this time period. On average, sample respondents smoked 18 cigarettes, or slightly less than one full pack, per day. A plurality of smokers (46%) had a monthly household income between ¥1000 and ¥3000 (US$150 to US$450). About a third of the study sample had a junior high school education, about a third had a high school education, and the remainder was split between a primary or tertiary education.

MULTIVARIATE RESULTS

The main study results are based on a conditional logit regression of cigarette tier prices on tier choice, controlling for wave, city, sex, age, income, education

Table 2:   Descriptive Statistics, 2006–2009

Variable Description	Mean	SD
Binary variables		
Male	0.963	—
Monthly household income: <¥1000	0.161	—
Monthly household income: ¥1000–2999	0.464	—
Monthly household income: ¥3000–4999	0.240	—
Monthly household income: ≥ ¥5000	0.134	—
Education: Primary school or less	0.125	—
Education: Middle school	0.327	—
Education: High school	0.358	—
Education: Beyond secondary school	0.190	—
Wave 1 (2006)	0.332	—
Wave 2 (2007–08)	0.365	—
Wave 3 (2009)	0.303	—
City: Beijing	0.172	—
City: Shenyang	0.138	—
City: Shanghai	0.224	—
City: Changsha	0.185	—
City: Guangzhou	0.142	—
City: Yinchuan	0.139	—
Continuous variables		
Age at Wave 1	50.8	12.3
Cigarette tier price, nominal	6.32	6.36
Cigarette tier price, real, in 2006 terms	6.24	6.30
Average daily cigarette consumption at Wave 1	17.7	10.8

Binary variables equal 1 if the description applies and 0 otherwise. The sample includes 3477 smokers and 8552 person-years, weighted based on the complex survey design.

and baseline cigarette intake. Table 3 shows the results of this regression. Own-tier price has a statistically significant negative effect on a smoker's choice of that tier. We consider the magnitude of the price effects in further detail below. Older smokers are significantly more likely to choose cheaper tiers. Smokers with low socioeconomic status — those with low income (below ¥1000) or low education (primary school or less) — are significantly more likely to buy from the cheapest tier, and, similarly, the probability of choosing a higher-priced tier increases with socioeconomic status. Baseline cigarette consumption is not consistently associated with tier choice, although the probability of choosing Tier 2 decreases with baseline consumption. Relative to smokers in Beijing,

Table 3:   Regression Results from Conditional Logit Model

	No Interaction	Interacted with Tier 2	Interacted with Tier 3	Interacted with Tier 4
Cigarette tier price	−0.095***			
	(0.015)			
Male		0.653***	0.717***	0.847**
		(0.177)	(0.264)	(0.420)
Age		−0.031***	−0.060***	−0.068***
		(0.006)	(0.006)	(0.007)
Income: ¥1000–2999		0.503***	1.086***	0.931***
		(0.114)	(0.152)	(0.193)
Income: ¥3000–4999		0.757***	1.872***	2.010***
		(0.167)	(0.203)	(0.238)
Income: ≥ ¥5000		1.183***	2.483***	3.073***
		(0.239)	(0.263)	(0.295)
Education: Middle school		0.467***	0.658***	0.430*
		(0.168)	(0.199)	(0.243)
Education: High school		0.545***	0.975***	0.981***
		(0.174)	(0.206)	(0.237)
Education: Beyond secondary		0.879***	1.511***	1.747***
		(0.218)	(0.258)	(0.282)
Cigarette consumption at Wave 1		−0.006	−0.143**	−0.009
		(0.005)	(0.006)	(0.007)
Wave 2		−0.165	−0.034	0.197
		(0.101)	(0.113)	(0.133)
Wave 3		0.006	0.242*	0.645***
		(0.113)	(0.134)	(0.147)
City: Shenyang		−0.186	−0.081	1.426***
		(0.180)	(0.209)	(0.303)
City: Shanghai		0.993***	3.462***	4.502***
		(0.271)	(0.274)	(0.363)
City: Changsha		1.257***	0.336	2.866***
		(0.197)	(0.236)	(0.311)
City: Guangzhou		0.644***	1.810***	1.454***
		(0.208)	(0.225)	(0.358)

(Continued)

Table 3:   (*Continued*)

	No Interaction	Interacted with Tier 2	Interacted with Tier 3	Interacted with Tier 4
City: Yinchuan		1.244***	0.459*	2.942***
		(0.207)	(0.249)	(0.314)
Constant		1.235***	0.832	−0.828
		(0.442)	(0.539)	(0.637)
Number of persons	3477			
Number of person-years	8552			
Number of observations	34208			

Robust standard errors, in parentheses, are clustered at the person level and weighted for survey sampling. The omitted category for categorical variables is: income below ¥1000, primary education and below, Wave 1 and Beijing. The model includes tier-specific constants.
Statistical significance: $^*p < 0.10$ $^{**}p < 0.05$ $^{***}p < 0.01$.

those in Shanghai and Guangzhou consistently have a greater likelihood of selecting a higher-priced tier (Tiers 2–4).

The magnitude of the average marginal effect of price on tier choice is described in Table 4. Panel A includes the net marginal price effects of moving in and out of a given tier, and Panel B includes the gross marginal price effects of moving out of a tier for those smokers who chose that given tier in Wave 1.

We start by describing the net price effects and then describe the gross price effects. If the price of Tier-1 cigarettes rose ¥1, then the net change in the probability of choosing Tier-1 cigarettes would decrease by 0.9% points (i.e., a negative own-price effect) and the net change in the probability of choosing other tiers would increase (i.e., a positive cross-price effect). Similarly, the average net own-price effects for Tiers 2–4 correspond to declines in the probability of using each respective tier by 1.9% points, 1.5% points and 0.9% points. A ¥1 increase corresponds to a 20% increase in the overall median cigarette price in our sample (¥5). Whereas on net trading up to a more expensive tier is more likely than downtrading among Tier-2 smokers, the reverse is true for Tier-3 smokers. In addition, we use the share of smokers within each tier (second-to-last row in Panel A of Table 4) to interpret the percentage change in the share choosing each tier as implied by that tier's net own-price effect (last row in Panel A of Table 4). Dividing the net own-price

Table 4: Average Marginal Price Effects on Switching Tiers

	Tier 1	Tier 2	Tier 3	Tier 4
Panel A. Net effects				
Median Tier-1 price	**−0.890**	0.640	0.200	0.070
	(0.012)	(0.010)	(0.003)	(0.001)
Median Tier-2 price	0.622	**−1.943**	0.857	0.426
	(0.010)	**(0.009)**	(0.008)	(0.006)
Median Tier-3 price	0.198	0.866	**−1.515**	0.450
	(0.003)	(0.008)	**(0.013)**	(0.010)
Median Tier-4 price	0.071	0.437	0.458	**−0.946**
	(0.001)	(0.006)	(0.010)	**(0.011)**
Number of person-year observations	8552	8552	8552	8552
Share of observations in Tier k	12.64%	44.68%	28.70%	13.99%
% change in share choosing Tier k, implied by net own-price effect	−7.04%	−4.35%	−5.28%	−6.76%
Panel B. Gross effects				
Median Tier-1 price	**−4.050**	0.169	0.154	—
	(0.056)	(0.004)	(0.005)	
Median Tier-2 price	2.775	**−0.552**	0.672	—
	(0.048)	**(0.006)**	(0.016)	
Median Tier-3 price	0.800	0.265	**−1.676**	—
	(0.028)	(0.004)	**(0.019)**	
Median Tier-4 price	0.474	0.118	0.850	—
	(0.020)	(0.003)	(0.015)	
Number of person-year observations	1236	4206	2522	—
Share of observations starting in Tier k	100.0%	100.0%	100.0%	—
% change in share choosing Tier k, implied by gross own-price effect	−4.05%	−0.55%	−1.68%	—

Average marginal price effects, reported as percentage points, are calculated from the conditional logit regression in Table 3. For each Tier k = (1, 2, 3, 4), bolded numbers denote the effect of median Tier-k price on the probability of choosing that same Tier k (i.e., the own-price effect), and unbolded numbers indicate the cross-effect of median Tier-k price on the probability of choosing Tier j ≠ k (i.e., the cross-price effect). Standard errors bootstrapped with 1000 repetitions are in parentheses. Net effects in Panel A, calculated on the full sample, capture the combination of movement into and out of a tier. Gross effects in Panel B, calculated for those starting in each given tier, capture movement out of a tier. The regression for the Tier-4 gross effects failed to converge due to a small sample.

effect for a given tier by the share of smokers within that tier, we calculate that ¥1 increase translates roughly into a 4–7% decrease in the net share choosing that tier, depending on the starting tier. The largest behavioural effects occur among smokers in the cheapest and the most expensive tiers.

The gross effect of tier-switching among those who used a given tier at baseline follows a similar pattern, although the magnitude of the marginal effects varies somewhat between the net and gross effects. If the price of Tier-1 cigarettes rose by ¥1, then smokers of Tier-1 cigarettes would be 4.1% points less likely to choose Tier 1 in subsequent waves. The gross own-price effects for Tiers 2 and 3 are about 0.6% points and 1.7% points. In other words, Tier-1 smokers are most likely to respond to the ¥1 price change. This is consistent with the fact that ¥1 represents a larger relative price change for a pack of inexpensive cigarettes from Tier 1 than for a pack of more expensive cigarettes from Tier 3. The added price sensitivity for Tier 1 holds when we look at how large this price effect is relative to the share of starting smokers in each tier (second-to-last row of Panel B in Table 4). The ¥1 increase translates into a 4% decrease in the gross share choosing Tier 1, compared with a 1–2% decrease for Tier-2 and Tier-3 smokers. Trading up is more common for Tier-2 smokers, similar to the net effects, whereas trading up and down appears to be equally common for the Tier-3 smokers.

We ran several sensitivity analyses to validate the association between price and tier choice (results not shown). We find some evidence that the relationship is not attributable to use of smuggled cigarettes. Among the subgroup of smokers who provided to the survey enumerators a pack with an authenticity label, which we assume to be indicative of a legally purchased pack, the price coefficient is of similar magnitude (−0.087) and statistically indistinguishable from the full sample (p = 0.61). The similarity between survey and retail price data also provides some suggestive evidence that smuggling and counterfeiting are not major concerns in our sample, because illicit tobacco use should lead the mean survey price to diverge from retail survey prices, which we do not find. The choice of sample composition — those individuals present in two or more waves — also did not affect the magnitude of the effect. Placing no restrictions on those included in the analysis (n = 10 020), the price coefficient is −0.075, insignificantly different from the restricted sample (p = 0.17). Likewise, restricting the sample to those present in all three waves (n = 4839) yields a price coefficient of −0.086, also insignificantly different from our final sample (p = 0.64).

DISCUSSION

Nearly 40% of smokers in our sample switched tiers across survey rounds, indicating that consumers are relatively flexible in brand choices and do not display strong loyalty to one brand variety. Brand choice appears to be sensitive to the price of cigarettes, controlling for each smoker's income and several other sociodemographic characteristics. We find that a ¥1 increase in the median price of a given tier would lead 4–7% fewer smokers to select that given tier, combining the net effect of smokers moving into and out of that tier. Isolating the gross effect of a ¥1 increase in the median price of a given tier on the probability of moving out of that tier, smokers who use cigarettes from the cheapest Tier 1 would be 4% less likely to select Tier 1 cigarettes following the price increase, whereas smokers of Tier-2 or Tier-3 cigarettes at Wave 1 would be only 1–2% less likely to select their starting tier. Thus, users of cheap cigarettes appear to be more sensitive to price increases when selecting a cigarette brand. To the extent that consumers can trade down to a cheaper brand while remaining within the same tier, our estimates may understate the degree to which price drives brand-switching. Overall, our findings underscore the role that tobacco pricing and tax policies can play in a consumer's brand decision and the degree to which consumers strategically switch brands.

The Chinese government influences retail cigarette prices by regulating their four constituent parts: the tax base (the allocation price), the value-added tax, profit margins for wholesalers and profit margins for retailers.[19] Current pricing regulations (of profit margins) may inadvertently promote downtrading to cheaper cigarettes among consumers. China permits more lucrative profit margins to wholesalers and retailers of higher-priced cigarettes than for lower-priced cigarettes (Table 1). These incentives likely contribute to China's large price spread. More importantly, if cigarette manufacturers and retailers are able to stimulate demand for higher-priced cigarettes through advertising and special promotions, then these practices facilitate the ability of smokers to trade down to cheaper cigarettes in times of economic hardship.

China's tax policy is a direct contributor to consumers' choice of cigarette brands. In China, cigarette taxes as a percentage of retail prices have held steady at roughly 40% in recent years,[23] compared with the World Health Organization's recommended benchmark of 70%.[24] Low excise taxes on cigarettes mean that consumers feel little financial pressure to reduce tobacco expenditures by quitting smoking. Rather, smokers have the ability to purchase cheap cigarettes. The composition of cigarette taxes is perhaps more important for brand-switching than the level of taxation. In particular, ad valorem taxes (assessed as a percentage of price) and specific taxes (assessed as a fixed amount per unit) have different effects on the incentives for consumers to choose relatively less expensive brands. An increase in a uniform ad valorem tax rate would leave unchanged the relative prices across tiers while increasing the absolute price difference. Since relative prices determine resource allocation in standard microeconomic theory, a uniform increase would not alter the gains to trading down to a cheaper brand. However, in China's tiered tax system, an increase in the ad valorem tax would increase the absolute price spread and the relative prices across tiers, effectively increasing the payoff to trading down to a cheaper brand. One would expect the probability of downtrading to increase with the payoff. Moreover, China's unusually large price spread for cigarettes serves as a positive moderator of the impact of ad valorem taxes, accentuating the payoff to downtrading. In contrast, a specific tax shrinks the per cent variance across tiers, reducing the payoff to switching to a relatively cheaper brand. Specific excise taxes are superior to ad valorem taxes in reducing the absolute share of cheap cigarettes that are available in a given market, likely reducing the degree to which consumers trade down and likely increasing the extent to which a tax increase induces consumers to quit smoking. These features of specific taxes are key to why experts have advocated a reliance on specific tobacco taxation.[24]

The current excise tax structure in China includes specific and ad valorem taxes.[7] However, the specific tax is a mere ¥0.06 per pack. In May 2009, China's State Tobacco Monopoly Administration officially raised the ad valorem tax rates to 56% of allocation prices for packs that have an allocation price of ¥7 or more, 36% on those costing less than ¥7 and an additional 5% tax applied to the wholesale price. However, the government directed the tobacco industry to absorb the tax increase, leaving retail prices unchanged.[11] Thus, the tax rates felt by consumers are far less than official rates indicate. Overall, China's tax structure does little to deter downtrading and may promote it through its reliance on ad valorem taxation.

Public health experts have encouraged the Chinese government to raise tobacco taxes as a way to increase cigarette prices and curb smoking rates.[25] Over the coming years, China is expected to follow these recommendations, in conjunction with its obligations under Article 6 of the Framework Convention on Tobacco Control, which covers price and tax measures for reducing the demand for tobacco products. Our study indicates that the design of the tax — namely ad valorem versus specific — will affect how consumers respond to the tax. The exact impact is difficult to quantify. Downtrading diminishes the price elasticity of demand to the extent that consumers' counterfactual response to the tax hike, in the absence of an ability to trade down, would be to quit smoking. In order to estimate the effect of a tax on consumer behaviour with and without downtrading, one would need to make assumptions about (1) the share of consumers who would smoke if allowed to trade down and who would quit otherwise, (2) the size and type of tax being imposed and (3) the differential impact of specific and ad valorem taxes on trading down. Our study can inform this third assumption, but we are not aware of any existing studies that address the probability of quitting under scenarios with and without downtrading. It is a topic worthy of future research.

Our study has several limitations. First, we characterised the degree of brand substitution across tiers, but we were unable to explore brand-switching within tiers. Second, we relied on self-reported prices, which could suffer from reporting bias (e.g., under-reporting the price due to use of illicit cigarettes). However, the similarity between self-reported and retail prices offers some evidence that any bias is likely to be small. Finally, our analyses do not take into account heterogeneity in smokers' preferences (e.g., by education and income category), although it is an area we plan to pursue in future research.

What this paper adds

- China's government is widely expected to raise cigarette tax rates in the next decade, but how Chinese consumers will respond to a cigarette price increase is not well understood.
- This paper describes for the first time how cigarette prices have influenced the cigarette brand choice of Chinese smokers.
- The discrete choice methodology offers a rigorous approach for identifying the impact of cigarette prices on purchasing behaviour.

ACKNOWLEDGEMENTS

We thank Qiang Li for access to the retail price data and Anne Chiew Kin Quah for administrative support. We also thank Frank Chaloupka for helpful comments and suggestions. All errors are our own.

Contributors JSW conceived and designed the study, analysed the data, interpreted the results, and drafted the manuscript. JL analysed the data, interpreted the results, and drafted the manuscript. TH conceived and designed the study and contributed to revisions of the manuscript. GTF supervised data collection and commented on an earlier draft of the manuscript. JY supervised data collection. All authors reviewed and approved the final manuscript. The corresponding author had full access to all data and final responsibility for the decision to submit the report for publication.

Funding JSW was supported by a grant from the US National Institute on Aging (T32-AG000246). TH was supported by a grant from the US Fogarty International Center (R01-TW05938). GTF was supported by a Senior Investigator Award from the Ontario Institute for Cancer Research and by a Prevention Scientist Award from the Canadian Cancer Society Research Institute. The ITC China Project was supported by grants from the US National Cancer Institute (R01-CA125116 and P01-CA138389), the Roswell Park Transdisciplinary Tobacco Use Research Center (P50-CA111236), the Canadian Institutes of Health Research (57897, 79551 and 115216), and the Chinese Center for Disease Control and Prevention.

Competing Interests None.

Patient Consent Obtained.

Ethics Approval The ITC China Surveys were cleared for ethics by Research Ethics Boards or International Review Boards at the University of Waterloo (Canada), Roswell Park Cancer Institute (USA), and the Chinese Center of Disease Control and Prevention.

Provenance and Peer Review Not commissioned; externally peer reviewed.

REFERENCES

1. Blecher EH, van Walbeek CP. Cigarette affordability trends: an update and some methodological comments. *Tob Control* 2009;18:167–75.

2. Li Q, Hyland A, Fong GT, *et al.* Use of less expensive cigarettes in six cities in China: Findings from the International Tobacco Control (ITC) China Survey. *Tob Control* 2011;19:i63–8.

3. Hyland A, Hibee C, Li Q, *et al.* Access to low-taxed cigarettes deters smoking cessation attempts. *Am J Public Health* 2005;95:994–5.

4. Chaloupka FJ, Warner KE. The economics of smoking. In: Culyer AJ, Newhouse JP, eds. *Handbook of health economics.* Vol. 1. 2000:1539–627.

5. International Agency for Research on Cancer. *Effectiveness of tax and price policies for tobacco control. Chapter 5.* Lyon, France: International Agency for Research on Cancer. 2011:137–200.

6. Gallet CA, List JA. Cigarette demand: a meta-analysis of elasticities. *Health Econ* 2003;12:821–35.

7. Hu T, Mao Z, Shi J, *et al. Tobacco taxation and its potential impact in China.* Paris: International Union Against Tuberculosis and Lung Disease, 2008.

8. Lance PM, Akin JS, Dow WH, *et al.* Is cigarette smoking in poorer nations highly sensitive to price? Evidence from Russia and China. *J Health Econ* 2004;23:173–89.

9. White JS, Hu T. How do Chinese smokers respond to changes in cigarette prices? Unpublished working paper. 2012.

10. Mao Z, Sung HY, Hu TW, *et al.* The demand for cigarettes in China. Chapter 7. In: Hu TW, ed. *Tobacco Control Policy Analysis in China.* Hackensack, NJ: World Scientific Publishing Co., 2008:129–57.

11. Huang J, Zheng R, Chaloupka F, *et al.* Price Responsiveness among Chinese Urban Adult Smokers: Findings from the ITC China Survey. *Presentation at World Conference on Tobacco or Health.* Singapore, 2012.

12. Evans WN, Farrelly MC. The compensating behavior of smokers: Taxes, tar, and nicotine. *RAND J Econ* 1998;29:578–95.

13. Tsai YW, Yange CL, Chen CS, *et al.* The effect of Taiwan's tax-induced increases in cigarette prices on brand-switching and the consumption of cigarettes. *Health Econ* 2005;14:627–41.

14. Hanewinkel R, Radden C, Rosenkranz T. Price increase causes fewer sales of factory-made cigarettes and higher sales of cheaper loose tobacco in Germany. *Health Econ* 2008;17:683–93.

15. Ohsfeldt RL, Boyle RG, Capilouto E. Effects of tobacco excise taxes on the use of smokeless tobacco products in the USA. *Health Econ* 1997;6:525–31.

16. Wangen KR, Biørn E. How do consumers switch between close substitutes when price variation is small? The case of cigarette types. *Spanish Economics Review* 2006;8:239–53.

17. White JS, Ross H. Do Smokers Undermine the Health Goals of Cigarette Taxes? Unpublished working paper. 2013.

18. Wu C, Thompson ME, Fong GT, *et al.* Methods of the International Tobacco Control (ITC) China Survey. *Tob Control* 2010;19:i1–5.

19. Gao A, Zheng R, Hu TW. Can increases in the cigarette tax rate be linked to cigarette retail prices? Solving mysteries related to the cigarette pricing mechanism in China. *Tob Control* 2012;21:560–2.

20. McFadden D. Conditional logit analysis of qualitative choice behavior. In: Zarembka P, ed. *Frontiers in Econometrics.* New York, NY: Academic Press 1973;105–42.

21. National Bureau of Statistics of China (2012a). Tobacco Consumer Price Index, 2006–2009. http://www.stats.gov.cn/tjsj/ (accessed 26 Nov 2012).

22. National Bureau of Statistics of China (2012b). Import Urban Resident Income Data, 2006–2009. http://www.stats.gov.cn/tjsj/ (accessed 26 Nov 2012).

23. Hu T, Mao Z, Shi J. Recent tobacco tax rate adjustment and its potential impact on tobacco control in China. *Tob Control* 2010;19:80–2.

24. World Health Organization. WHO Technical Manual on Tobacco Tax Administration. Geneva, Switzerland, 2011.

25. World Health Organization. WHO Supports Increasing Prices for Tobacco in China. 2012. Press Release. http://www2.wpro.who.int/china/media_centre/press_releases/PR_20120314.htm/(accessed 21 Apr 2012).

The Heterogeneous Effects of Cigarette Prices on Brand Choice in China: Implications for Tobacco Control Policy*

Jing Li, Justin S. White, Teh-wei Hu, Geoffrey T. Fong
and Jiang Yuan

ABSTRACT

Background China has long kept its tobacco taxes below international standards. The Chinese government has cited two rationales against raising tobacco tax, namely, the unfair burden it places on low-income smokers and the ability of consumers to switch to cheaper brands.

Objective This study examines how different socioeconomic subgroups of Chinese smokers switch brands in response to cigarette price changes.

Methods We model smokers' choice of cigarette tier as a function of tier-specific prices. We examine heterogeneous responses to prices by estimating mixed logit models for different income and education subgroups that allow for random variation in smokers' preferences. We use data from three waves of the longitudinal International Tobacco Control China Survey, collected in six large Chinese cities between 2006 and 2009.

---

*Published in *Tob Control*, 2015; 0:1–8. doi: 10.1136/tobaccocontrol-2014-051887 (April 8, 2015).

Findings Low-income and less educated smokers are considerably more likely to switch tiers (including both up-trading and down-trading) than are their high-socioeconomic status (SES) counterparts. For those in the second-to-lowest tier, a ¥1 ($0.16, or roughly 25%) rise in prices increases the likelihood of switching tiers by 5.6% points for low-income smokers and 7.2% points for less educated smokers, compared to 1.6% and 3.0% points for the corresponding high-SES groups. Low-income and less educated groups are also more likely to trade down compared to their high-SES counterparts.

Conclusions Only a small percentage of low-income and less educated Chinese smokers switched to cheaper brands in response to price increases. Hence, the concern of the Chinese government that a cigarette tax increase will lead to large-scale brand switching is not supported by this study.

INTRODUCTION

China ratified the Framework Convention on Tobacco Control (FCTC) in 2005. A key provision of the FCTC is to raise the price of cigarettes through taxation, in recognition of smokers' sensitivity to cigarette prices. Nevertheless, the Chinese government has been reluctant to raise cigarette prices through taxation, evidenced by the fact that the government enacted a complicated reclassification of cigarette price levels and tax rates in 2009, but explicitly banned producers from passing the tax increase onto consumers.[1] One barrier with respect to raising the cigarette tax is the belief among some Chinese political leaders that cigarette taxes place an unfair burden on low-income smokers.[2]

Another barrier to further tax increase is that some Chinese political leaders have questioned the effectiveness of using cigarette taxes to control tobacco use. They believe that given the very wide price range of cigarettes in China — from ¥2 to more than ¥100 (¥1 = $0.16) per pack — smokers can easily switch to cheaper brands in response to a tax-induced price increase, thus maintaining the same cigarette consumption. Government officials frequently invoke this argument in private conversations. While this reasoning may seem compelling, no existing studies have quantified the magnitude of such switching behaviour, to our knowledge.

In an earlier paper using several waves of the ITC (International Tobacco Control) China Survey data, we addressed the effect of cigarette prices on brand switching among the entire smoking population and found the magnitude of switching to be moderate but non-trivial: a ¥1 change in the price of cigarettes alters the tier choice of 4–7% of smokers, depending on the starting tier.[3] However, we did not examine the possible differential effects of price changes among different socioeconomic groups of the population, which is particularly important for policymakers concerned about the relative financial burden of increased taxes on low-income smokers. The purpose of this paper is to provide empirical evidence about the effect of cigarette prices on the magnitude of brand switching among various socioeconomic groups of smokers in China and to address the implications for tobacco tax policy for tobacco control.

The rest of this paper is organised as follows. Section 2 details the methods, including data, measures and analytical strategy. Section 3 presents the descriptive and multivariate results. Section 4 discusses the implications of our findings for tobacco control policy in China and other countries.

METHODS

Data

Data for this study come from the ITC China Survey, an individual-level, longitudinal survey of smoking behaviour among adults in China. Our analytical sample is derived from the first three waves of the ITC China Survey, fielded in 2006, 2007–2008 and 2009, in six cities of China: Beijing, Shanghai, Guangzhou, Shenyang, Changsha and Yinchuan. These cities are diverse and broadly representative of China's urban areas. A multistage clustered sampling method was employed at the city level, yielding approximately 800 respondents per city and wave.

As the objective of this paper is to track smokers' brand-switching behaviour over time, we restricted our sample to 4632 continuing smokers who participated in at least two waves of the ITC China Survey. After applying further restrictions described in detail below, our final analytic sample included 3477 individual smokers who constituted 8552 person-years. Overall retention in our final sample is 82%.

Measures

Our dependent variable is the market segment (i.e., grade or tier) in which a smoker's chosen brand falls in a given wave. We construct this variable using information on the most recent purchase of cigarettes reported by each smoker. Specifically, respondents were asked to provide the brand family and variety, total amount paid and quantity bought for cigarettes that they most recently purchased for themselves. Cigarettes in a brand family are produced by the same manufacturer. Meanwhile, one brand family often contains several brand varieties that are of different prices. For instance, under one brand family such as 'Double Happiness', there are different brand varieties such as 'Hard' and 'Soft'. Often, different brand varieties with the same brand family can belong to different price tiers.

We followed several steps in assigning a tier to each smoker's last purchased cigarettes. First, we computed the per-pack cigarette price by dividing the total amount paid by number of packs bought (the vast majority of cigarette packs in China contain 20 cigarettes each). For quantity reported in cartons, we multiplied the number of cartons by 10 to obtain the number of equivalent packs. Second, we validated the self-reported information using retail price data collected in the same six cities at the same time as Wave 3. Overall, the retail prices were extremely similar to average brand-specific prices from the Wave-3 survey data. For the eight most frequently purchased brand varieties, the city-level average retail price and the city-level median self-reported survey price were identical in all markets for five varieties and differed by less than ¥0.5 (4% or less) for the remaining three varieties.

Third, we assigned a unique code to each brand variety using the Universal Product Code on the barcode of each pack. For cases in which the preassigned code was missing and a descriptive name was entered in the 'Other' variety and family fields, we manually assigned a brand variety code based on the names provided by respondents. Based on this procedure, we successfully assigned a brand variety code to 78% of all observations, which consist of 3477 individual smokers as our final sample. Next, we calculated the median price for each brand variety in each city at each wave as the basis for assigning price tiers.

Finally, we sorted brand varieties into price tiers using the six-grade classification system of allocation prices (analogous to producer prices) that the Chinese government uses to assess excise taxes. For purposes of consistency, we use the same classification for all three waves despite the fact that there was a minor adjustment of cigarette classification and profit margins by the Chinese government in 2009[4] (we provide more explanation of this below). Since the purpose of sorting brand varieties into price tiers is to divide the cigarette market into meaningful segments from the perspective of consumers instead of producers, only the retail prices matter. We converted allocation prices into

Table 1: Cigarette Retail Prices in China by Tier, 2009

Grade	Tier	Retail Price (¥/pack)	Producer Profit (%)	Retail Profit (%)	Smoker-years (N)	Smoker-years (%)
1		[29.76, ∞)	51.5	15	59	0.7
2	1	[18.95, 29.76)	40.8	15	150	1.8
3		[8.97, 18.95)	33.3	15	955	11.3
4	2	[5.15, 8.97)	33.3	10	2345	27.7
5	3	[2.65, 5.15)	25	10	3830	45.3
6	4	[0, 2.65)	17.6	10	1114	13.2
					8453	100

Note: Retail price ranges are calculated according to the formula (Gao *et al.*[5]): Retail Price = Allocation Price × (1 + Producer π) × (1 + Retail π) × (1 + VAT), where π denotes profit and VAT is the value-added tax. The ranges for profits come from Gao, Zheng and Hu (2011). For retail price ranges, a bracket denotes a closed interval and a parenthesis denotes an open interval. Tiers 4–6 are combined for analysis due to small cell sizes. Cell counts and proportions are survey weighted. The unweighted sample size is 8552 person-years from 3477 smokers.

retail prices using a standard formula reported in Gao *et al.*[5] Table 1 shows the retail price ranges for each tier. Since data were sparse at high prices, we combined the three most expensive grades (grades 1, 2 and 3) into a single tier (Tier 1). Hence, our final classification included four price tiers. In the rest of the paper, we refer to the tiers with the most expensive cigarettes as Tier 1 and those with the cheapest cigarettes as Tier 4. We assigned each observation to a price tier based on the range into which its by-city median brand variety price fell. For instance, if a smoker in Beijing purchased a soft pack of White Sand in Wave 1, which has a median price of ¥5, then we assigned this person-year observation to Tier 3.

Our key independent variable is the market price per pack for each tier in a given wave. We used nominal prices, as China's cigarette price index indicates that inflation was negligible during the study period. In order to account for any recall and reporting biases in the self-reported price measures, we used the median price of all cigarette brands that fall into a given price tier as that tier's market price. Variation in relative median prices of tiers comes from two sources. First, the six cities surveyed are located in different provinces of China, and each province has cigarette factories that produce their own set of brands.[6] Each city thus has a slightly different composition of brands offered to local consumers. Accordingly, brands not manufactured locally are transported from other cities and provinces and their prices are influenced by random fluctuations in the costs of transportation and handling, which is plausibly unrelated to local demand.

Second, in 2009, the Chinese government implemented an adjustment in its tobacco tax structure in order to raise revenue, which effectively decreased the profit margin on the lower-priced cigarettes relative to higher-priced cigarettes.[4] The government prohibited the resulting tax increase from being passed on directly to smokers; therefore, the retail price of a given cigarette brand was left unchanged.[2] However, the tobacco industry responded by decreasing the production of low-priced cigarettes that became less profitable and increasing the production of high-priced cigarettes that became more profitable. This leads to a change in distribution of production, which in turn decreased the availability of cheap cigarettes (i.e., those with a per-pack price below ¥3) nationwide and raised the median price in the lower tiers, as within each tier the more expensive brands have become more available compared to the less expensive ones.[4] This is meaningful to our study as our price measure is not the retail price of any particular brand of cigarettes, but is the median price of all cigarette brands in a given tier, which is more influenced by the *distribution* of prices on the cigarette market. In addition, the tax adjustment likely affected different cities differently because of the heterogeneity in the composition of brands produced across local markets.

Our regressions control for a variety of demographic characteristics of smokers: gender, age, income, education and average number of cigarettes consumed per day at baseline. Gender, income and education are coded as categorical variables, whereas age and baseline consumption are coded as continuous variables. We constructed socioeconomic subgroups for income and education, as detailed below. We also added city and wave fixed effects to control for time-invariant and city-specific unobserved factors as well as for aggregate trends that are constant across cities. As brand-specific advertising and marketing are banned in China, these are unlikely to bias our results.

Analytical Strategy

Our estimation approach uses a mixed logit model that describes smokers' choices among different tiers of cigarettes. The value in this particular approach in comparison with other discrete choice models such as conditional logit is its ability to allow for random variation in smokers' tastes for different brands and estimation of individual-specific parameters.[7] Instead of assuming a fixed model parameter (e.g., coefficient on price) for each individual in the data and producing an estimate for that parameter, the mixed logit model allows the assumption that the parameter of interest is a random variable following a certain distribution, most commonly assumed to be normal, in the population. Accordingly, the mixed logit model produces estimates of the mean as well as the SD of the parameter of interest that is assumed to be random, which capture the average magnitude of the random variable as well as the extent of its variation in the sample.

In setting up the model, we assume that a utility-maximising smoker faces a choice among J alternative cigarette quality tiers in each of T choice situations. The utility that smoker i obtains from tier choice j in choice situation t is a function of observed and unobserved factors:

$$U_{ijt} = \alpha_i \, p_{ijt} + \beta'_j X_{it} + \omega_{ij} + \varepsilon_{ijt}$$

where p_{ijt} is the market price of tier j faced by smoker i at time t; α_i is the smoker-specific coefficient on price; X_{it} is a vector of observed smoker characteristics including wave and city fixed effects; β_j is a vector of coefficients specific to tier j on observed smoker characteristics; ω_{ij} represents the time-invariant unobserved component of smoker-specific utility from cigarette tier j; and ε_{ijt} captures time-varying unobserved factors that affect smoker i's choice and is assumed to be distributed i.i.d. extreme value. Smoker i maximises utility by choosing the cigarette quality tier that yields the highest utility: $Pr(Tier_{it} = k) = Pr(U_{ikt} > U_{ijt}, \text{ for all tiers } j \neq k)$.

In implementing the mixed logit model, we assume that the price coefficient α_i and tier-fixed effects ω_{ij} are random variables that take on different values across smokers ('random coefficients'), reflected by the i subscript, whereas the vector of coefficients on observed characteristics are assumed to be fixed ('fixed coefficients'). We think these are reasonable assumptions given that different smokers may respond to cigarette price changes differently (even within a group with similar socioeconomic status (SES)), and smokers are also likely to have varying tastes over cigarettes in a given quality tier even after controlling for observable characteristics.

We estimate the model by simulating the log-likelihood function. Since the model allows for an individual-specific price parameter α_i and tier dummies ω_{ij}, the estimated parameters consist of the means as well as the SDs of the distributions of α_i and ω_{ij} across our sample of smokers.

In performing the estimation, we divided the sample in two ways for the purpose of investigating the heterogeneous effects of prices on cigarette tier choice across SES subgroups. Note that although the mixed logit model allows for heterogeneous price coefficients across individuals, it does not permit direct analysis on how price effects vary by SES if estimated on the full sample only. The survey asked respondents to report their monthly household income in one of four categories: below ¥1000, ¥1000–2999, ¥3000–4999 and at or above ¥5000. In addition, there were four categories of educational attainment: primary school or less, at least some middle school, at least some high school and beyond high school. In our analysis, we defined the high-income group as having monthly income at or above ¥3000 (approximately $483), compared to a low-income group of less than ¥3000. Independently, smokers were classified as more educated if they had at least some high school education and less educated if they had no high school education. Although our choice of SES cut-offs is constrained by the information available in the survey data, these cut-offs appear to accord with the distribution of income and education at the national level. Mean monthly household income among urban residents in China was about ¥3600 in 2007.[8] In addition, about 60% of Chinese citizens had received education beyond middle school in 2010.[9] We estimated the model first for the full sample and then for these four subgroups separately.

Given that the coefficients from a mixed logit model are difficult to interpret directly, we also estimated the average marginal effects of cigarette tier prices, which is the change of probability in choosing a given cigarette tier resulting from a ¥1 increase in the median price of that tier, accounting for movement into and out of a given tier (ie, net effects). We computed bootstrapped SEs for the average marginal effects, using 1000 repetitions and clustering at the individual level. Again, marginal effects were computed both for the full sample and by SES subgroup to facilitate analysis of the heterogeneous response to price changes.

RESULTS

Sample Characteristics

Table 2 presents the descriptive statistics of the smokers in the full sample and by subgroup. Using the monthly income threshold of ¥3000, about 62% of smokers in our sample had low incomes. In addition, approximately

Table 2:　Descriptive Statistics, 2006–2009

Variable Description	Full Sample	Low Income	High Income	Less Educated	More Educated
Binary variables					
Male	0.963	0.954	0.978	0.940	0.982
Monthly household income					
< ¥1000	0.161	0.258	—	0.239	0.097
¥1000–2999	0.464	0.742	—	0.518	0.420
¥3000–4999	0.240	—	0.642	0.179	0.291
≥ ¥5000	0.134	—	0.358	0.065	0.191
Education					
Primary school or less	0.125	0.156	0.072	0.277	—
Middle school	0.327	0.390	0.222	0.724	—
High school	0.358	0.348	0.376	—	0.653
Beyond high school	0.190	0.106	0.331	—	0.347
Continuous variables					
Age at baseline	50.8	51.4	49.6	54.1	48.0
	[12.3]	[12.4]	[12.4]	[12.3]	[11.8]
Cigarette tier price					
Nominal	6.32	5.35	7.92	5.16	7.26
	[6.36]	[4.30]	[8.54]	[4.11]	[7.60]
Real, in 2006 terms	6.24	5.29	7.82	5.10	7.18
	[6.30]	[4.25]	[8.47]	[4.05]	[7.54]
Average daily cigarette	17.7	17.9	17.0	18.6	16.8
consumption at baseline	[10.8]	[11.3]	[9.75]	[11.3]	[10.3]
Number of smoker-years	8453	5288	3166	3820	4633

Note: Coefficients are means of each variable by sample. Binary variables equal 1 if the description applies and 0 otherwise. SDs for continuous variables are in square brackets. The numbers of smoker-years in each column are weighted based on the complex survey design.

55% smokers had some high school and thus belong to the more educated subgroup. Over 96% of smokers are male across all subsamples. The average price of cigarettes purchased is ¥6.32 in the full sample, which is virtually unchanged after adjusting for inflation. As expected, on average, high-SES smokers purchase more expensive cigarettes than their low-SES counterparts. In addition, respondents across all subsamples smoked slightly less than one full pack per day. Although average cigarette price appears to be quite low, the high cigarette intake and relatively low income of Chinese smokers suggest that cigarette consumption likely accounts for a non-trivial portion of household expenditures. Based on observed cigarette consumption and prices, a rough estimate is that an average smoker with a monthly household income of ¥3000 would spend 5.6% of this income on cigarettes.

Regression Estimates

Table 3 presents the coefficient estimates from the mixed logit model for the full sample. These coefficients may be loosely understood as the effects of different factors on the likelihood of choosing a particular cigarette tier.[10] The mean coefficient on price is negative and significant, suggesting that as cigarette tier price increases, the probability of purchasing cigarettes in that tier significantly diminishes. There is substantial heterogeneity in the value that smokers attach to cigarettes in a given tier, as indicated by the large, statistically significant SDs of the coefficients on the alternative-specific constants that is, on the tier dummies.

In general, one would expect cigarettes in more expensive tiers to have higher quality and to be more attractive to smokers, holding all else constant. This appears to be the case as the tier dummy coefficients decrease steadily from Tier 2 to 4. Interestingly, Tier 1 has a lower mean coefficient estimate than Tier 2. There are two possible explanations for why, all else equal, smokers may attach greater value to cigarettes in Tier 2 than in Tier 1. First, cigarettes in the highest tier are most commonly purchased as gifts in China,[1] therefore the majority of smokers may not value cigarettes in this tier as much when purchased for self-consumption. Second, most consumers of very expensive cigarettes may use them as a type of 'status good',[11] that is, to signal that person's economic and social status to others, rather than for normal everyday consumption, which would limit the occasions in which very expensive cigarettes may be needed or yield very high utility.

Smoker characteristics also have significant effects on the choice of cigarette brand tiers as illustrated by the coefficients on demographic covariates in Table 3. The probability of choosing more expensive tiers decreases significantly with age. In addition, smokers with a low income and less education are far more likely to purchase cigarettes in lower tiers. The substantial heterogeneity in brand choice by SES in the full model motivates further analysis by subgroup.

Table 3: Regression Results from Mixed Logit Model

	No Interaction	Interacted with Tier 1	Interacted with Tier 2	Interacted with Tier 3
Random coefficients				
Cigarette tier price — mean	−0.314***			
	(0.049)			
Cigarette tier price — SD	0.221***			
	(0.031)			
Constant — mean		4.565***	5.101***	2.558***
		(1.006)	(0.777)	(0.631)
Constant — SD		1.119***	1.159***	1.524***
		(0.256)	(0.129)	(0.105)
Fixed coefficients				
Male		0.961	0.803**	0.760***
		(0.614)	(0.340)	(0.240)
Age		−0.087***	−0.075***	−0.033***
		(0.009)	(0.008)	(0.007)
Income: < ¥1000		−3.644***	−2.692***	−1.009***
		(0.385)	(0.308)	(0.291)
Income: ¥1000–2999		−2.509***	−1.544***	−0.512**
		(0.310)	(0.267)	(0.262)
Income: ¥3000–4999		−1.265***	−0.648**	−0.386
		(0.324)	(0.286)	(0.281)
Income: ≥ ¥5000 (omitted)				
Education: Primary school and below (omitted)				
Education: Middle school		0.496	0.499**	0.678***
		(0.340)	(0.243)	(0.212)
Education: High school		1.337***	1.204***	0.899***
		(0.330)	(0.254)	(0.225)
Education: Beyond high school		2.505***	2.039***	1.277***
		(0.380)	(0.310)	(0.260)
Cigarette consumption at Wave 1		−0.011	−0.016**	−0.005
		(0.009)	(0.008)	(0.007)
Wave fixed effects	Yes			
City fixed effects	Yes			
Number of persons	3477			
Number of person-years	8552			
Number of observations	34 208			

Note: Robust SEs, in parentheses, are clustered at the person level and weighted for survey sampling. The omitted category for categorical variables is: income above ¥5000, primary education and below, Wave 1 and Beijing. The model includes tier-specific constants. 'Interacted with Tier x' means the coefficient is on the interaction term between the variable listed in the first column with Tier x (x = 1, 2, 3, 4), as mixed logit model allows variables that vary over choice alternatives, which is similar to conditional logit. Significance: *p < 0.10, **p < 0.05, ***p < 0.01.

Marginal Effects of a Price Change by SES Subgroup

In order to further interpret the magnitudes of brand-switching, we calculate the average marginal effect of each cigarette price, defined as the effect of a ¥1 price increase for a given tier on the predicted probability of choosing that tier. This ¥1 increment corresponds to a 20% increase in the median price of cigarettes in our sample (¥5).

Table 4 shows the marginal own-price effects for the full sample and by SES subgroup. For each tier, increasing the price by ¥1 while holding the prices

Table 4:   Marginal Own-price Effects: Full Sample and by Subgroup

	Tier 1	Tier 2	Tier 3	Tier 4
Full Sample	−1.445***	−3.268***	−4.484***	−2.665***
	(0.023)	(0.029)	(0.017)	(0.030)
	[−10.33]	[−11.39]	[−10.04]	[−21.08]
Subgroup analysis				
Low-income smokers	−1.308***	−3.203***	−5.648***	−3.733***
(Income < ¥3000)	(0.023)	(0.041)	(0.021)	(0.041)
	[−13.52]	[−13.90]	[−11.11]	[−22.68]
High-income smokers	−1.141***	−1.862***	−1.601***	−0.753***
(Income ≥ ¥3000)	(0.020)	(0.014)	(0.016)	(0.015)
	[−5.37]	[−4.87]	[−4.66]	[−12.12]
Z-score of between-group difference	5.48	30.95	153.29	68.26
p > |z|	<0.0001	<0.0001	<0.0001	<0.0001
Less educated smokers	−1.374***	−3.994***	−7.171***	−4.872***
(Less than high school)	(0.034)	(0.067)	(0.032)	(0.065)
	[−15.62]	[−17.08]	[−14.27]	[−27.73]
More educated smokers	−1.353***	−2.713***	−2.967***	−1.520***
(At least some high school)	(0.029)	(0.027)	(0.024)	(0.027)
	[−7.17]	[−8.05]	[−7.53]	[−19.01]
Z-score of between-group difference	0.470	17.73	105.1	47.62
p > |z|	0.64	<0.0001	<0.0001	<0.0001

Note: Each row of coefficients comes from a separate regression. Average marginal own-price effects and SEs are reported as percentage points. Bootstrapped SEs derived from 1000 repetitions are in parentheses. The percentage change in the share of smokers choosing Tier k is in square brackets; this is derived from the own-price effect and the percentage of observations in Tier k at baseline.
Significance: *$p < 0.10$, **$p < 0.05$, ***$p < 0.01$.

of other tiers constant is associated with a statistically significant decrease in the probability of choosing that tier. For the full sample of smokers, from the most expensive to cheapest tier, the own-price effect is a decrease of 1.45% points, 3.27% points, 4.48% points and 2.67% points. Correspondingly, the share of smokers in each tier decreases by 10.3%, 11.4%, 10% and 21.1% in response to a ¥1 increase in tier price. These magnitudes imply that smokers in the middle two tiers are most likely to respond to a price change by switching to another tier. In part, this reflects the constraints that consumers on the extremes face: smokers of discount brands (Tier 4) have no ability to trade down and smokers of premium brands (Tier 1) have no ability to trade up.

Marginal own-price effects for the full sample of smokers mask important heterogeneity in price responses by SES subgroup. Rows 2–7 of Table 4 present the marginal own-price effects for each subgroup: low-income, high-income, less educated and more educated smokers. In all cases but one, low-income and less educated smokers are far more likely to switch tiers compared to their high-SES counterparts, as demonstrated from the p values of z-scores of subgroup differences in marginal propensity of switching. Low-income or less educated smokers who initially purchased cigarettes in Tier 3 are most responsive to prices: a ¥1 rise in prices increases the likelihood of switching tiers by 5.6% points (11.1% decrease in tier share) for low-income smokers and 7.2% points (14.3% decrease in tier share) for less educated smokers, compared to 1.6% (4.7% decrease in tier share) and 3% points (7.5% decrease in tier share) for the corresponding high-SES groups. By contrast, the probability of brand switching for those who start in Tier 1 seems to be quite small and relatively stable across SES group. Even though the p value still shows significant difference between high-income and low-income smokers in Tier 1, the z-score of between-group difference is much smaller compared to other tiers. Again, this would be consistent with gift-giving and the consumption of status goods as explained earlier, as these special purposes make it less likely that cigarettes in lower tiers will serve as good substitutes for premium cigarettes, hence lowering the likelihood of brand switching out of Tier 1.

In addition to own-price effects, the mixed logit estimates provide the cross-price effects of, say, a price change in Tier 2 on the probability of choosing Tiers 1, 3 and 4. The relative size of the cross-price effects for higher versus lower tiers provides a measure of the share of smokers who traded up to a higher quality tier versus the share who traded down to a lower quality tier following a ¥1 increase in tier price. This procedure is only informative for the middle

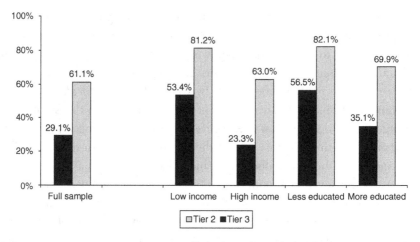

Fig 1:　Percentage of switchers who trade down.

tiers for which individuals are able to substitute bidirectionally. Figure 1 shows the percentage of switchers who trade down by tier and subgroup. Among switchers, those who purchased cigarettes in Tier 3 at baseline are on average more than twice as likely to trade up to more expensive cigarettes (70.9%) than to trade down to the cheapest tier (29.1%). In contrast, those who purchased cigarettes in Tier 2 at baseline are less inclined to trade up (38.9%) than to trade down (61.1%).

There are large differences across subgroups in the percentage of switchers who trade down as opposed to trading up. In all cases, the low-income and less educated groups are more likely to trade down. Among switchers who purchased Tier 3 cigarettes at baseline, 53.4% of low-income smokers traded down compared to 23.3% of high-income smokers. The parallel estimates of down-trading for switchers who purchased Tier 2 cigarettes at baseline are 81.2% of low-income smokers and 63% of high-income smokers. The differences by schooling are also stark: for switchers starting in Tier 3, 56.5% of less educated smokers trade down versus 35.1% of more educated smokers; and for those starting in Tier 2, 82.1% of less educated smokers trade down versus 69.9% of more educated smokers.

DISCUSSION

We find large heterogeneity in the brand-switching behaviour of smokers in response to price changes. We find that SES and the starting tier are important sources of heterogeneity in how smokers respond to price changes. Specifically, low-income and less educated smokers are far more likely to engage in brand switching compared to high-income or more educated workers: on net, approximately 11% to 23% low-income smokers and 14% to 28% less educated smokers in a given tier switch to an alternative tier in response to a ¥1 increase in the price of the starting tier, whereas only about 5% to 12% high-income and 7% to 19% more educated smokers do so. The difference in marginal effects is statistically significant across subgroups for each tier except between less and more educated smokers in Tier 1.

In addition, the likelihood of switching from the low and middle tiers is much higher than the likelihood of switching from the highest tier, especially for low-income and less educated smokers. Across all models, low-income and less educated groups are more likely to trade down compared to their high SES counterparts. Based on the results from Table 4 and Figure 1, a ¥1-increase in the price of a given tier induces 1.3–3% of all low-income smokers and 1.4–4.1% of all less educated smokers to switch to a cheaper tier, whereas only 1–1.2% high-income smokers and 1–1.9% more educated smokers do so.

It is worth noting that from the mixed logit model, the estimates of SDs for the random variables — in this case the coefficients on price and tier fixed effects — are all statistically significant and quite large in magnitude, suggesting that there is substantial variation in smokers' sensitivity to price and taste for different cigarette tiers, thereby justifying the use of mixed logit model. In comparison, conditional logit model (results not shown) tends to underestimate the magnitude of the price coefficient by restricting it to be fixed across smokers.

One caveat in interpreting the results of our study is that we only examine brand switching across tiers. To the extent that smokers may switch brands within a given tier, our results may still underestimate the true extent of brand-switching among Chinese smokers.[3] However, since the three lowest tiers in our classification in which smokers are more sensitive to price all have reasonably narrow price ranges (approximately ¥3, or $0.5), it is unlikely that our method would severely underestimate the magnitude of brand-switching, especially for low-income and less educated smokers who are much more likely to consume cigarettes in one of the three lowest tiers.

Overall, we find evidence of only moderate magnitude of smokers switching to less expensive tiers in response to price increase, as shown in our back-of-envelope calculation (Paragraph 2 of this section). This has at least three implications for tobacco control policy. First, brand switching does not appear to be a valid reason for the Chinese government to avoid raising tobacco taxes. Given the relatively small magnitude of trading down among different SES subgroups of smokers, we would expect this factor to have minimal impact on the effectiveness of a cigarette tax increase. Second, our study indicates that brand switching would be most likely to occur following tax adjustments that alter the relative prices of cigarettes across tiers. The 2009 tax reform, though it left brand-specific retail prices unchanged, set higher allowable profit margins for premium brands. This shifted production toward premium brands and decreased the availability of cheaper cigarettes, thus moving the peak of the distribution of cigarette prices to the right. When low-priced cigarettes are no longer available, smokers who view higher-priced cigarettes as a reasonable substitute will be likely to trade up, as evidenced by the data. Future tax reform needs to take this behaviour into account by equalising the cross-tier incentives of cigarette manufacturers to produce one price tier versus another, thereby discouraging both up-trading and down-trading. Third, there may be an important role for public education aimed at shattering the high-status image of high-end cigarettes. The denormalisation of smoking in Western countries began with the high-SES population. If the same holds true in China, then we would expect that, as increasing numbers of wealthier Chinese smokers quit smoking, the demand for premium cigarettes should decline. The result would be a compression of the price distribution. More research is needed to understand the motivations of Chinese smokers for consuming high-end cigarettes.

Furthermore, the fact that low-income or less educated smokers are more likely to engage in brand switching highlights how price-sensitive these groups are. It is unlikely that these subgroups would be willing to sacrifice a significant portion of income just to maintain consumption of cigarettes from which they derive limited utility. A carefully designed tax reform, namely one that discourages brand switching, holds promise for decreasing cigarette consumption among low-SES smokers, rather than shouldering them with a greater financial burden. As we have also argued in previous work,[3] an increase in ad valorem tax rates, imposed as a percentage of price, would further amplify the cigarette price spread, creating more incentives for smokers to trade down to cheaper cigarettes. By contrast, a specific excise tax, a fixed amount per unit, would reduce differences in relative tier prices, thereby discouraging down-trading. A specific excise tax is the preferred policy instrument for curbing brand switching, yet China's current excise tax is an insignificant ¥0.06 ($0.01) per pack. The overall tobacco tax rate in China is only 40–46% of retail prices, far below the WHO standard of 70%.[3] Hence there is ample scope for China to raise its specific excise tax on tobacco.

We believe that the issue of the potential regressivity of taxes is an important one. While we are not aware of any studies documenting a differential adverse impact of taxation on low-SES groups in China, studies in other settings have raised this concern.[12] It is an empirical question whether tobacco taxes in China are regressive. To the extent that they are, we believe that transfer payments may be an effective policy instrument for the Chinese government to address the differential financial and health burdens from smoking experienced by low-SES groups. In light of the country's recent experience with healthcare reform, the revenues from increased tobacco taxes may be used as subsidies on insurance premiums or healthcare expenditures, to be directed toward socioeconomically disadvantaged groups.

Finally, our case study of China's cigarette market may also be instructive for other countries in Asia. India, Vietnam, Indonesia and certain other countries have a large share of low-income smokers and the availability of cheap tobacco products. Our findings regarding brand switching by SES group in China suggest that an increase on excise taxes for tobacco products may also be effective in other contexts that share similar characteristics to the tobacco market as China.

What this paper adds

- This paper is the first to examine brand choice behaviour by socioeconomic status of smokers in China.
- The finding is important in assessing the two rationales commonly cited by the Chinese government against tax increase, namely, the unfair burden it places on low-income smokers and the ability of consumers to undo a tax's health effects by switching to cheaper brands.
- Mixed logit model offers a flexible and rigorous approach for identifying the impact of cigarette prices on purchasing behaviour.

ACKNOWLEDGEMENTS

The authors work has benefitted from input from Frank Chaloupka, Ben Handel, Jiun-Hua Su and Ken Train. The authors thank Qiang Li for access to the retail price data and Anne C K Quah for administrative support.

Contributors JL analysed the data, interpreted the results and drafted the manuscript. JSW conceived and designed the study, analysed the data, interpreted the results and contributed to drafting and revisions of the manuscript. T-wH conceived and designed the study and contributed to drafting and revisions of the manuscript. GTF supervised data collection and commented on an earlier draft of the manuscript. JY supervised data collection. All authors reviewed and approved the final manuscript. The corresponding author had full access to all data and final responsibility for the decision to submit the report for publication.

Funding JSW was supported by a grant from the US National Institute on Aging (T32-AG000246). T-wH was supported by a grant from the US Fogarty International Center (R01-TW009295). GTF was supported by a Senior Investigator Award from the Ontario Institute for Cancer Research and by a Prevention Scientist Award from the Canadian Cancer Society Research Institute. The ITC China Project was supported by grants from the US National Cancer Institute (R01-CA125116 and P01-CA138389), the Roswell Park Transdisciplinary Tobacco Use Research Center (P50-CA111236), the Canadian Institutes of Health Research (57897, 79551 and 115216) and the Chinese Center for Disease Control and Prevention.

Competing interests None.

Patient consent Obtained.

Ethics approval The ITC China Surveys were cleared for ethics by Research Ethics Boards or International Review Boards at the University of Waterloo (Canada), Roswell Park Cancer Institute (USA) and the Chinese Center of Disease Control and Prevention.

Provenance and peer review Not commissioned; externally peer reviewed.

REFERENCES

1. Hu T, Lee AH, Mao Z. WHO framework convention on Tobacco control in China: barriers, challenges and recommendations. *Glob Health Promot* 2013;20:13–22.

2. Hu T, Mao Z, Shi J. Recent tobacco tax rate adjustment and its potential impact on tobacco control in China. *Tob Control* 2010;19:80–2.

3. White JS, Li J, Hu T, *et al.* The effect of cigarette prices on brand-switching in China: a longitudinal analysis of data from the ITC China Survey. *Tob Control* 2014;23:i54–i60.

4. Zheng R, Gao S, Hu T. Tobacco tax and tobacco control: global experience and its application in China. *Finance Trade Econ* 2013;3:44–53.

5. Gao S, Zheng R, Hu T. Can increases in the cigarette tax rate be linked to cigarette retail prices? Solving mysteries related to the cigarette pricing mechanism in China. *Tob Control* 2011;21:560–2.

6. Tong E, Tao M, Xue Q, *et al.* China's tobacco industry and the world trade organization. In: Hu T, ed. *Tobacco control policy analysis in China.* Hackensack, NJ: World Scientific Publishing Co., 2008:211–244.

7. Train KE. *Discrete choice methods with simulation.* New York, NY: Cambridge University Press, 2009.

8. National Bureau of Statistics of China (2014). Urban Resident Income Data, 2007. http://data.stats.gov.cn/workspace/index?m=hgnd (accessed 20 Apr 2014).

9. National Bureau of Statistics of China (2011). 2010 Sixth National Population Census Report. http://www.stats.gov.cn/tjsj/tjgb/rkpcgb/qgrkpcgb/201104/t20110428_30327.html (accessed 20 Apr 2014).

10. Train KE, Winston C. Vehicle choice behavior and the declining market share of US automakers. *Int Econ Rev* 2007;48:1469–96.

11. Chen X, Zhang X. Costly posturing: relative status, ceremonies and early child development. Unpublished working paper. 2011.

12. Colman GJ, Remler DK. Vertical equity consequences of very high cigarette tax increases: if the poor are the ones smoking, how could cigarette tax increases be progressive? *J Policy Anal Manage* 2008;27:376–400.

8

The Epidemic of Cigarette Gifting: A Social Barrier to Tobacco Control in China

Xiulan Zhang, Steve Lin and Teh-wei Hu

ABSTRACT

Context One of the challenges China faces in implementing tobacco control policies is to change the social norm, especially the culture and behaviors surrounding cigarette gift giving.

Objectives To develop evidence for the tobacco control policy initiative issued in China at the end of 2013.

Methods Analysis of data from a national survey on tobacco utilization that contains information on cigarette gift exchanges, conducted by the China Bureau of Statistics in 31 provinces of China from October to November 2005.

Participants A national representative random sample of 171,924 persons aged 15 years or older from 23,000 urban and 37,000 rural households. The sample was based on the 2005 Census. Of the sample, 171,876 people had valid data, and 43,457 smokers reported information on cigarette gift exchanges.

Results 19.11% of Chinese smokers reported receiving cigarettes as gifts, 9.02% of smokers gave cigarettes to others, and over 23% of the smokers had either received or given cigarettes as gifts. Given that the survey was not conducted during the country's highest gift-giving occasion, the Chinese New Year, the rate of cigarette gift exchange could actually be much higher than these figures suggest. The highest smoking prevalence (39.08%) and the highest rate of cigarette gifting (36.05%) were reported by smokers working for government agencies. The multivariate results show urban smokers were more likely to receive cigarette gifts (Odds = 1.13). Male smokers were less likely to receive cigarette gifts than female smokers (Odds = 0.88). Smokers between the ages of 15 to 19 were more likely to receive or give cigarette gifts. Higher educated and high-income smokers were more likely to receive cigarette gifts, and smokers with a high school education level were more likely to send cigarettes to others.

Conclusions Tobacco control measures should be aimed at changing the cigarette gifting culture and behavior in China. Targeting government officials, higher educated and high-income people will help remove the social barriers to implementing tobacco control in China. In November, 2013, China's State Council released regulation against giving cigarette as gift to government officials. This was a major step for the Chinese government to change the social norm from using cigarette as a means of gift giving. It should help to remove one of the social barriers of tobacco control.

INTRODUCTION

China's 356 million current smokers consume the largest share of the world's cigarettes each year. In addition, 740 million Chinese people are exposed to secondhand smoke in public places, workplaces, and indoors, which means that 80% of China's population are first or secondhand smokers.[1] Annually, over one million of China's smokers die from smoking-related diseases. In addition, hundreds of thousands of people die or get ill from secondhand smoke.[2] Treating tobacco-related diseases is putting a heavy burden on China's healthcare financing system.[3,4] High medical expenses and spending on cigarettes[5] is especially hard on China's poor households and can crowd out the investment in children's education.[6] Without reducing China's smoking prevalence, it is estimated that by the year 2030, two million people will die each year from smoking.[7,8]

Studies have indicated that social dimensions related to tobacco products and social exchanges of cigarettes by youth contribute to their smoking behavior.[9–12] A study of adolescent behavior in China revealed that a high rate of accepting cigarettes offered by friends results in a 5–17 times higher probability of being a lifetime or current smoker.[13]

The importance of abolishing the social exchange of cigarettes by youth led public health researchers to study cultural practices associated with tobacco use.[14,15] Their studies found that mainstream smoking cessation approaches were challenged by China's culture of gifting and sharing cigarettes, a tradition rooted in its history and social relationships.[13,16,17,19] In China, smoking serves as a social function,[19] and tobacco serves as a social currency.[16–18]

The practice of cigarette gifting and sharing among the Chinese is maintained even when they migrate to other nations.[15]

The custom of cigarette gifting was explored by transnational tobacco companies when they entered cigarette markets in China.[20,21] A review of internal tobacco industry documents by Chu, Jiang and Glantz[21] found that British American Tobacco (BAT) and Philip Morris (PM) used marketing research firms to gain understanding of the social norms of cigarette sharing and gifting in China. Firms identified marketing strategies to reinforce cigarette gifting during key holiday occasions and to expand cigarette gifting to Chinese people outside China.

The flow of gifts has long been an integral part of Chinese culture and social fabric, and it helps in acquiring power, status, and resources.[22,23] Not only is smoking still a very acceptable social behavior, but sharing cigarettes and exchanging cigarette gifts also have been considered important in social networking and building relationships.[24,25] Because cigarette gifting normalizes smoking across Chinese society and promotes the social acceptability of tobacco, it has been one of the major barriers to carrying out tobacco control in China.[25] Cigarette gifting promotes economic returns to the tobacco industry and establishes smoking as a role model for the rest of the society.

This study is the first to analyze the social norm of cigarette gifting. It aims to help Chinese policymakers effectively implement the recent gifting regulation for government officials enacted as part of the anti-corruption movement of the new administration.

METHODS

The 2005 National Tobacco Use Survey (NTUS) was conducted by the National Bureau of Statistics. It was designed to collect representative nationwide data on cigarette smoking behavior and the use of tobacco products for people in China over the age of 15. The survey adopted the 2005 one percent population survey sampling framework. It surveyed 37,000 rural and 23,000 urban households between the end of October and the middle of November 2005. NTUS contains data on basic household characteristics and detailed individual smoking behaviors. Household variables include family size, total income, and total expenses. Individual variables within the family include age, gender, marital status, educational level, occupation, smoking history, age started smoking, number of cigarettes smoked per day, type of cigarettes, price of cigarettes, favorite brand (domestic or imported), tobacco consumption costs, and the demand for low cost cigarettes. Most important, the survey contains information on cigarette exchanges. The total effective sample size is 171,876 individuals in 59,845 households with 52,617 current smokers.

Of the total 52,617 current smokers, 47,557 smoke cigarettes, and 43,457 of them filled out cigarette purchasing and gifting questionnaires. The specific questions asked in the survey are: (1) "In the past three months, how many packages of cigarettes have you bought or obtained?" (2) "Of the total cigarettes, how many packages did you buy, and how many packages were gifts from others?" (3) "Of the total cigarettes purchased or obtained, how many packs did you smoke, and how many packs did you give to others?" If the total cigarettes the person received from others in the past three months were greater than zero, then the gift cigarettes received variable was coded as one; otherwise, the variable was coded as zero. If the total cigarettes the person gave to others in the past three months were greater than zero, then the gift cigarettes gave variable was coded as one; otherwise, the variable was coded as zero. If the person received or gave cigarettes, then the cigarette exchange variable was coded as one. If the person neither received nor gave cigarettes, then the cigarette exchange variable was coded as zero. All statistical analyses were conducted using SAS 9.3.

RESULTS

The total prevalence of smoking in 2005 was 30.6%. The rural smoking rate was higher than the urban rate; 56.7% of males smoked, while only 2.56% of females smoked. People under the age of 30 had a lower smoking prevalence. People with a high school education had the highest smoking rate compared with people with higher and lower educational levels. Over one third of managers, business owners, farmers, and workers were smokers, and nearly 40% of the people working for government agencies were smokers. No significant differences were found in smoking prevalence among income groups, but smoking rates differed across areas of residence.

With respect to the cigarette gifting behaviors, 19.11% of smokers received cigarette gifts, 9.02% of smokers gave cigarettes to others, and over 23% of the smokers had either received or given cigarettes as gifts, but only about 5% of the smokers had both received and given cigarettes to others. Table 1 presents the socio-demographic characteristics of the full sample and the sub-sample of current smokers with cigarette gifting information. The highest rate of cigarette gifting was reported by smokers working for government agencies; more one third of them either received or gave cigarettes as gifts. The second highest rate of cigarette gifting was observed among the teachers, doctors, and military personnel.

Table 2 presents the results from the multivariate logistic regressions on receiving, giving, or exchanging cigarette gifts. Variables included in the model are urban versus rural, male versus female, 5-year age groups, educational level, marital status, occupation, working for the government or not, income level, and region where smokers live.

The results show that urban smokers were more likely to receive than give cigarette gifts, and the total cigarette exchange rate is about the same between rural and urban smokers. Male smokers were less likely to receive cigarette gifts than female smokers. Smokers between ages 15 to 19 and older than age 70 were more likely to receive cigarette gifts, and the older the smokers, the less likely they will give cigarettes to others.

The higher the educational level, the more likely a smoker is to receive cigarette gifts, and smokers with high school education level were more likely to send cigarettes to others. No significant differences were found in cigarette gifting by marital status, but significant differences were found across occupations. Business owners, farmers, workers, and not employed smokers were less likely to receive cigarettes, and workers, farmers, and not employed also were less likely to send cigarettes to others.

Smokers working for government agencies were more likely to receive cigarette gifts, and the higher the receivers' income level, the more likely they were to receive or give cigarettes gifts. Cigarette gift exchange behaviors differed by living areas, with smokers living in the central China region reporting more cigarette gift exchanges.

We further examined the perception of the brands that smokers bought for gifts. The question was: Of all the brands you have smoked, please choose the three best brands. For each of the three brands, what was the price, and what was the assessment? The assessment included five items on taste, three items on reputation, packaging, and price, two items on harm, and six items

Table 1:   Socio-demographic Characteristics of the Samples

| Variable | Full Sample N = 171,876 | | Sample with Cigarette Gifting Information (Smokers Only) N = 43,457 | | | | |
	% Sample	Prevalence (%)	% Sample	% Receiving	% Giving	% Receiving or Giving	% Receiving and Giving
Total	100	30.61	100	19.11	9.02	23.26	4.87
Location							
Urban	34.56	28.74	36.61	24.08	8.59	27.78	4.88
Rural	65.44	31.60	63.39	16.24	9.26	20.64	4.86
Gender							
Male	51.82	56.70	94.01	19.00	9.06	23.17	4.89
Female	48.18	2.56	5.99	20.80	8.38	24.61	4.58
Age Group							
15–19	10.47	3.23	0.69	20.86	11.59	26.82	5.63
20–24	9.59	15.39	3.63	20.16	9.70	23.53	6.34
25–29	8.09	26.96	6.65	18.83	10.45	23.81	5.47
30–34	9.47	32.72	10.57	17.50	9.82	22.26	5.05
35–39	11.25	36.44	14.39	18.32	9.93	22.74	5.52
40–44	12.11	38.58	16.68	19.14	9.99	23.78	5.35
45–49	9.22	38.79	12.62	18.58	9.70	23.10	5.18
50–54	9.84	39.12	13.09	18.90	8.17	22.73	4.34
55–59	6.64	39.58	8.59	20.17	7.98	23.86	4.28
60–64	4.82	38.06	5.42	19.66	6.41	22.68	3.40
65–69	3.52	38.22	3.81	19.67	5.49	22.21	2.96
>=70	4.98	30.41	3.84	24.31	5.69	26.65	3.35
Educational Level							
Less than middle school	27.71	30.84	24.53	16.73	7.78	20.49	4.01
Middle school	39.07	32.72	42.11	15.76	8.47	20.00	4.24
High school	22.17	28.48	22.34	22.13	10.60	26.85	5.88
College and above	11.05	26.88	11.02	31.08	10.63	34.59	7.12
Marital Status							
Never Married	21.64	12.96	6.63	20.03	9.06	23.65	5.45
Married	74.08	35.59	89.50	19.06	9.10	23.29	4.87

(Continued)

Table 1:   (*Continued*)

Variable	Full Sample N = 171,876		Sample with Cigarette Gifting Information (Smokers Only) N = 43,457				
	% Sample	Prevalence (%)	% Sample	% Receiving	% Giving	% Receiving or Giving	% Receiving and Giving
Divorced/ Widowed	4.28	33.72	3.88	18.75	6.88	21.78	3.86
Occupation							
Manager	7.69	38.54	11.04	31.44	11.26	35.48	7.21
Teacher/ Doctor/ Military Personnel	2.28	25.52	2.17	31.95	13.16	35.88	9.24
Worker/ Farmer	57.15	34.94	62.39	15.43	8.24	19.42	4.26
Business Owner	5.04	41.61	7.47	19.10	12.78	26.25	5.64
Retired/ Freelancer	9.40	30.42	10.18	23.33	7.98	26.81	4.50
Student/not employed	14.81	7.98	4.05	19.89	6.59	22.50	3.98
Other	3.63	26.44	2.71	26.36	11.48	31.38	6.46
Working for Government Agency							
Yes	3.89	39.08	5.81	32.73	10.30	36.05	6.97
No	96.11	30.27	94.19	18.27	8.94	22.47	4.74
Income Level							
Under poverty line	3.87	29.21	3.11	15.19	5.19	17.33	3.04
101–200% poverty line	15.83	30.84	15.07	14.64	7.28	17.83	4.09
201–300% poverty line	20.78	30.50	20.39	15.91	8.07	20.02	3.96
>300% poverty line	59.52	30.68	61.43	21.47	9.95	25.96	5.45
Region							
North	11.10	33.68	12.25	16.13	6.20	19.46	2.87
Northeast	8.59	34.19	8.84	13.41	4.63	15.70	2.34
East	26.79	28.51	26.41	19.15	8.25	23.53	3.88
Central	28.35	26.99	24.56	29.38	13.40	34.80	7.98
Southwest	15.02	36.13	17.71	11.83	7.25	15.09	3.99
Northwest	10.14	31.73	10.23	15.46	10.69	20.09	6.05

Table 2:   Odds Ratio of Cigarette Gifting

Variable	Receiving (incl. Giving)		Giving (incl. Receiving)		Receiving or Giving		Receiving and Giving	
	Beta Estimates	OR (95% CI)	Beta Estimate	OR (95% CI)	Beta Estimate	OR (95% CI)	Beta Estimate	OR (95% CI)
Urban (vs rural)	0.119***	1.13 (1.05 to 1.21)	−0.352***	0.70 (0.64 to 0.77)	0.048	1.05 (0.98 to 1.12)	−0.424***	0.65 (0.58 to 0.74)
Male (vs female)	−0.128**	0.88 (0.79 to 0.98)	−0.085	0.92 (0.79 to 1.07)	−0.129**	0.88 (0.80 to 0.97)	−0.085	0.92 (0.76 to 1.12)
Age Group (vs older than age 70)								
15–19	−0.018	0.98 (0.70 to 1.38)	1.011***	2.75 (1.74 to 4.36)	0.258	1.29 (0.94 to 1.78)	0.651**	1.92 (1.03 to 3.57)
20–24	−0.196*	0.82 (0.67 to 1.01)	0.670***	1.96 (1.44 to 2.66)	−0.077	0.93 (0.76 to 1.13)	0.676***	1.97 (1.33 to 2.91)
25–29	−0.367***	0.69 (0.59 to 0.82)	0.623***	1.86 (1.44 to 2.42)	−0.165*	0.85 (0.73 to 0.99)	0.411**	1.51 (1.08 to 2.12)
30–34	−0.414***	0.66 (0.57 to 0.77)	0.553***	1.74 (1.36 to 2.22)	−0.228**	0.80 (0.69 to 0.92)	0.365**	1.44 (1.05 to 1.98)
35–39	−0.362***	0.70 (0.60 to 0.81)	0.562***	1.76 (1.38 to 2.23)	−0.210**	0.81 (0.71 to 0.93)	0.462***	1.59 (1.16 to 2.17)
40–44	−0.308***	0.74 (0.64 to 0.85)	0.574***	1.78 (1.40 to 2.25)	−0.149*	0.86 (0.75 to 0.99)	0.433**	1.54 (1.13 to 2.10)
45–49	−0.345***	0.71 (0.61 to 0.82)	0.549***	1.73 (1.36 to 2.21)	−0.190**	0.83 (0.72 to 0.95)	0.418**	1.52 (1.11 to 2.08)

50–54	-0.271***	0.76 (0.66 to 0.88)	0.394***	1.48 (1.17 to 1.89)	-0.165*	0.85 (0.74 to 0.97)	0.285*	1.33 (0.97 to 1.82)
55–59	-0.192**	0.83 (0.71 to 0.96)	0.368**	1.45 (1.13 to 1.85)	-0.107	0.90 (0.78 to 1.04)	0.283*	1.33 (0.96 to 1.83)
60–64	-0.228***	0.80 (0.68 to 0.93)	0.120	1.13 (0.86 to 1.48)	-0.179*	0.84 (0.72 to 0.97)	0.018	1.02 (0.72 to 1.45)
65–69	-0.266***	0.77 (0.65 to 0.91)	-0.047	0.96 (0.71 to 1.29)	-0.238**	0.79 (0.67 to 0.93)	-0.134	0.88 (0.59 to 1.30)
Educational Level (vs less than middle school)							
Middle school	-0.078*	0.93 (0.86 to 0.99)	-0.041	0.96 (0.87 to 1.06)	-0.073*	0.93 (0.87 to 0.99)	-0.044	0.96 (0.84 to 1.09)
High school	0.114**	1.12 (1.03 to 1.22)	0.161**	1.17 (1.05 to 1.31)	0.110**	1.12 (1.03 to 1.21)	0.243***	1.28 (1.10 to 1.48)
College and above	0.277***	1.32 (1.18 to 1.48)	0.128	1.14 (0.97 to 1.34)	0.220***	1.25 (1.12 to 1.39)	0.336***	1.40 (1.14 to 1.73)
Marital Status (vs divorced/widowed)							
Never Married	0.048	1.05 (0.87 to 1.26)	-0.113	0.89 (0.69 to 1.16)	0.003	1.00 (0.84 to 1.19)	-0.074	0.93 (0.66 to 1.31)

(Continued)

Table 2: (Continued)

Variable	Receiving (incl. Giving)		Giving (incl. Receiving)		Receiving or Giving		Receiving and Giving	
	Beta Estimates	OR (95% CI)	Beta Estimate	OR (95% CI)	Beta Estimate	OR (95% CI)	Beta Estimate	OR (95% CI)
Married	0.070	1.07 (0.94 to 1.22)	0.095	1.10 (0.90 to 1.34)	0.089	1.09 (0.97 to 1.24)	0.056	1.06 (0.82 to 1.37)
Occupation (vs other)								
Manager	0.024	1.02 (0.88 to 1.20)	−0.110	0.90 (0.72 to 1.11)	−0.018	0.98 (0.85 to 1.14)	−0.036	0.97 (0.73 to 1.27)
Teacher/Doctor/Military Personnel	0.066	1.07 (0.87 to 1.31)	−0.087	0.92 (0.70 to 1.21)	−0.005	1.00 (0.82 to 1.21)	0.043	1.04 (0.75 to 1.46)
Worker/Farmer	−0.487***	0.61 (0.53 to 0.71)	−0.510***	0.60 (0.50 to 0.73)	−0.516***	0.60 (0.52 to 0.68)	−0.559***	0.57 (0.45 to 0.73)
Business Owner	−0.359***	0.70 (0.59 to 0.82)	−0.034	0.97 (0.78 to 1.20)	−0.237**	0.79 (0.68 to 0.92)	−0.273*	0.76 (0.57 to 1.01)
Retired/Freelancer	−0.225**	0.80 (0.69 to 0.93)	−0.171	0.84 (0.68 to 1.05)	−0.233***	0.79 (0.68 to 0.92)	−0.147	0.86 (0.65 to 1.14)
Student/not employed	−0.300***	0.74 (0.62 to 0.89)	−0.462***	0.63 (0.48 to 0.82)	−0.370***	0.69 (0.58 to 0.82)	−0.366**	0.70 (0.49 to 0.98)
Working for a government agency (vs not working for the government)								
Work for a government agency	0.178***	1.20 (1.08 to 1.33)	−0.066	0.94 (0.80 to 1.10)	0.136**	1.15 (1.04 to 1.27)	0.010	1.01 (0.84 to 1.22)

Income Level (vs under poverty line)												
101–200% poverty line	−0.030	0.97 (0.82 to 1.15)		0.361***	1.44 (1.11 to 1.86)		0.044	1.05 (0.89 to 1.22)		0.321*	1.38 (0.99 to 1.93)	
201–300% poverty line	0.015	1.02 (0.86 to 1.20)		0.437***	1.55 (1.20 to 2.00)		0.136*	1.15 (0.98 to 1.34)		0.246	1.28 (0.92 to 1.78)	
>300% poverty line	0.277***	1.32 (1.13 to 1.54)		0.627***	1.87 (1.46 to 2.40)		0.380***	1.46 (1.26 to 1.70)		0.518***	1.68 (1.22 to 2.31)	
Region (vs North)												
Northeast	−0.205***	0.82 (0.72 to 0.92)		−0.239**	0.79 (0.65 to 0.95)		−0.239***	0.79 (0.70 to 0.88)		−0.138	0.87 (0.67 to 1.14)	
East	0.246***	1.28 (1.17 to 1.40)		0.341***	1.41 (1.23 to 1.60)		0.278***	1.32 (1.22 to 1.43)		0.351***	1.42 (1.18 to 1.71)	
Central	0.819***	2.27 (2.08 to 2.47)		0.871***	2.39 (2.11 to 2.71)		0.836***	2.31 (2.13 to 2.50)		1.092***	2.98 (2.50 to 3.55)	
Southwest	−0.248***	0.78 (0.70 to 0.87)		0.222**	1.25 (1.08 to 1.44)		−0.202***	0.82 (0.74 to 0.90)		0.402***	1.50 (1.23 to 1.83)	
Northwest	0.0640	1.07 (0.95 to 1.19)		0.667***	1.95 (1.68 to 2.26)		0.154**	1.17 (1.05 to 1.29)		0.856***	2.36 (1.92 to 2.89)	

(Significant level: *** <0.001, ** <0.05, and * <0.10).

Table 3:   Perceptions and Evaluations of the Brands for Gifts (N = 10323)

Assessment	Yes (%)	No (%)	Not Sure (%)
Prefer cigarette that tastes strong	45.47	44.31	10.23
Prefer cigarette that tastes moderate	72.28	19.78	7.94
Prefer cigarette that tastes mild	72.76	19.02	8.22
Prefer cigarette that the throat feels smooth	79.49	12.25	8.26
Prefer cigarette that smell good	74.41	15.38	10.21
Prefer cigarette that has a good reputation	50.03	20.51	29.46
Prefer cigarette that is beautifully packaged	47.76	37.37	14.86
Prefer cigarette that is reasonably priced	56.56	28.22	15.21
Prefer cigarette that has low tar	68.57	20.22	11.21
Prefer cigarette that has adopted high technology to lower the harms	26.84	19.70	53.46
Prefer cigarette that is suitable for people under age 40	52.63	21.34	26.03
Prefer cigarette that is suitable for the elderly	48.63	24.95	26.42
Prefer cigarette that is suitable for men	74.18	10.36	15.46
Prefer cigarette that is suitable for women	19.50	49.56	30.94
Prefer cigarette that is suitable for self-social status	60.57	24.80	14.64
Prefer cigarette that is suitable for gifts	46.56	36.71	16.73

regarding their suitability for specific groups. For each item, the assessment category included yes, no, or not sure. In the sample, 10,107 smokers either received or gave cigarette gifts, and 10,323 brands were rated by the 10,107 smokers.

Table 3 lists the smokers' perceptions and evaluations of the brands they bought for gifts. The results show that when smokers bought cigarettes as gifts, they preferred those cigarettes that taste moderate or mild, throat feels smooth, or smells good. Reputation, packaging, and price also were considerations in buying cigarette gifts. More than half of the respondents considered low tar content when purchasing, but only about a quarter of the people knew whether the cigarettes they bought as gifts were manufactured with technology to lower their harm level.

We conducted a factor analysis and retained one factor, with "yes" coded as 1, "no" or "not sure" coded as zero. We first included variables describing taste, reputation, price, and packaging, awareness of the harm, and the

Table 4: Results of the Factor Analysis on Brands for Gifts

Variable	Standardized Scoring Coefficients	Standardized Scoring Coefficients
Prefer cigarette that tastes strong	−0.013	−0.034
Prefer cigarette that tastes moderate	0.151	0.216
Prefer cigarette that tastes mild	0.161	0.237
Prefer cigarette that the throat feels smooth	0.156	0.227
Prefer cigarette that smell good	0.168	0.234
Prefer cigarette that has a good reputation	0.177	0.222
Prefer cigarette that is beautifully packaged	0.177	0.214
Prefer cigarette that is reasonably priced	0.023	0.024
Prefer cigarette that has low tar	0.144	0.207
Prefer cigarette that has adopted high technology to lower the harms	0.109	0.149
Prefer cigarette that is suitable for people under age 40	0.170	
Prefer cigarette that is suitable for the elderly	0.103	
Prefer cigarette that is suitable for men	0.144	
Prefer cigarette that is suitable for women	0.104	
Prefer cigarette that is suitable for self-social status	0.056	
Prefer cigarette that is suitable for gifts	0.154	

perception for gifts, and then we took out the perception variables and ran the model again. The standardized scoring coefficients are presented in Table 4.

The results of the factor analysis show that when smokers decided to buy cigarette as gifts, they preferred those cigarettes that taste moderate or mild, throat feels smooth, or smells good. Reputation and packaging also were important when considering cigarettes as gifts. Low tar was favored, which suggests that many smokers are aware of the harmful effect of smoking.

Smokers considered price in the brands they bought for gifts. The average price of a pack of cigarettes they themselves smoked was 4.24 RMB, while the average price for cigarettes they purchased as gifts was 9.11 RMB, more than twice the price of the cigarettes they smoked.

Chinese gift giving practices are common at "key gift giving festivals", which are the Chinese New Year and the Mid-Autumn Festival.[20,21] In the

Table 5:   Monthly Sales of Cigarettes (in Billions of Packs)

Year	During Chinese New Year	% Higher than Average	During Mid-autumn Festival	% Higher than Average	Average of the Other Months
2003	9.22	29.68%	7.77	9.28%	7.11
2004	9.31	22.99%	8.28	9.38%	7.57

Data source: NBS 2005 NTUS data report.

1990s, transnational tobacco companies made a big effort to promote cigarette gifting in China. British American Tobacco (BAT) promoted its brand by specifically targeting the Chinese New Year, and Philip Morris (PM) targeted its brand for gifting during the Mid-Autumn Festival.[21] Cigarette sales statistics confirmed the literature that during the Chinese New Year, the total packs of cigarettes sold was 29.68% higher in 2003, and 22.99% higher in 2004 than the average monthly sales for the non-major holiday months as shown in Table 5. The national statistics showed the monthly sales during the Mid-Autumn festival were over 9% higher than the average non-major holiday months.

DISCUSSION

This is the first detailed analysis of China's cigarette gifting behaviors based on national data; however, the data did not collect cigarette gift exchange information from nonsmokers. Moreover, the survey collected data that included both non-major holiday months and the month with the Mid-Autumn Festival, but not the month with the Chinese New Year. Thus the gifting prevalence rate estimated here is likely lower than the actual rate as many people exchange cigarette gifts during the Chinese New Year. A regional survey in east China conducted in 2010 by the China Center for Disease Control reported over 50% of the respondents planned to buy cigarettes as gifts for the Chinese New Year.[26] Another study reported 45% of Beijing residents reported they would send cigarette as gifts during Chinese New Year.[27]

This study finds that 23.26% of the smokers in the survey actually exchanged cigarette gifts from August to October. If we take into consideration the difference between average monthly cigarette sales and sales during the Chinese New Year, which are 23% to 30% higher than the average, the prevalence of cigarette gift exchange rate could be much higher than reported here.

This study has several implications for tobacco control policies. In addition to the MPOWER policy package proposed by WHO in 2008, which includes Monitor (M) tobacco use and prevention policies, Protect (P) people from tobacco smoke, Offer (O) help to quit tobacco use, Warn (W) about the dangers of tobacco, Enforce (E) bans on tobacco advertising, promotion and sponsorship, and Raise (R) taxes on tobacco,[28] tobacco control policies should combine culturally specific and effective approaches with the conventional methods. Social norm change is essential for China, especially in reducing cigarette sharing and gifting.[25]

This study finds that even though the cigarette gifting rates are lower because of the survey period, about a quarter of smokers have either received or/and given cigarettes as gifts. As cigarette gifting is common on the "key gifting occasions", public campaigns and anti-smoking education should make more effort on these key occasions, such as the Chinese New Year and the Mid-Autumn Festival.

The study reveals a striking phenomenon, which is that not only do government officials have the highest smoking prevalence, but they also have the highest rate of engaging in cigarette gifting exchanges, mainly as the receivers of cigarettes. Tobacco control advocates have done a remarkable job convincing Chinese leaders to stop cadres and officials from smoking in public places, and the national policy was issued at the end of 2013.[29] In addition, as part of the anti-corruption movement, officials are banned from receiving gifts, including cigarettes and alcohol. Under China's political top-down system, these new policies are a major step toward removing the social barriers to tobacco control in China. They should have a demonstrative effort of discouraging cigarette gift giving as a medium of exchange among the general public. It is crucial to enforce this policy, especially to involve the general public in monitoring the implementation of the policy, which not only can help change the behavior of the government officials with respect to exchanging cigarette gifts, but also can educate the public about this bad social norm.

According to the survey data, many smokers have some understanding of the harmfulness of smoking and are aware of this when they pick up the brands as gifts.[26] Therefore, messages should be developed that make it clear that giving cigarettes to the elderly is not good for their health, but rather may lead to illness and death, as older people in China are more likely to receive cigarettes as gifts.

This study shows that female smokers and young smokers in China are more likely to receive cigarette gifts than male smokers. Changing the gifting behavior for females and youth should be a priority. There also are significant regional differences in cigarette gifting, with the central and eastern regions of China having the highest prevalence. Anti-smoking campaigns should target these areas more.

As for choosing specific cigarette brands as gifts, price was not an important factor in the factor analysis, but packaging and reputation were. The China Advertisement Law began to solicit public comments in February 2014. We hope this law will stop the promotion of cigarettes, which should reduce cigarette gift exchange behavior.

Smokers with higher educational levels and higher income are more likely to give and receive cigarette gifts, and urban smokers are more likely to receive cigarette gifts. Because China is developing and urbanizing rapidly, because more people live in the cities, get richer, and have more education, tobacco control policies could be compromised if the social norm of cigarette giving is not changed.

In November, 2013, China's State Council released regulation against giving cigarette as gift to government officials. This was a major step for the Chinese government to change the social norm from using cigarette as a means of gift giving. It should help to remove one of the social barriers of tobacco control.

REFERENCES

1. Liu B-Q, Peto R, Chen Z-M, *et al.* Emerging tobacco hazards in China: Retrospective proportional mortality study of one million deaths. British Medical Journal 1998; 317:1411–1422.
2. Yang L, Sung HY, Mao ZZ, Hu TW. Economics costs attributable to smoking in China: update and an 8-year comparison, 2000–2008. Tobacco Control 2011; 20:266–72.
3. Yang L, Mao ZZ, Hu TW. The economic cost of smoking and the potential medical care cost savings by raising tobacco tax, High Level Policy Conference on Tobacco Taxation and Tobacco Economy, 13 November 2013, Beijing, China.
4. HU TW, Mao Z, Liu Y, de Beyer J, One M. Smoking, standard of living, and poverty in China. Tobacco Control 2005; 14:247–250.

5. Wang H, Sindelar JL, Busch SH. The impact of tobacco expenditure on household consumption patterns in China. Social Science and Medicine 2006; 62: 1414–1426.

6. Liu YL, Rao KQ, Hu TW, Sun Q, Mao ZZ. Cigarette smoking and poverty in China. Social Science and Medicine 2006; 63:2784–2790.

7. Quan G, Smith KR, Hammond SK, Hu TW. Disease burden of adult lung cancer and ischemic heart disease from passive tobacco smoking in China. Tobacco Control 2007; 16:417–422.

8. Shafey O, Eriksen M, Ross H, Mackay J. *The Tobacco Atlas.* 3rd ed. Atlanta, GA: American Cancer Society; 2009.

9. Harrison PA, Fulkerson JA, Park E. The relative importance of social versus commercial sources in youth access to tobacco, alcohol, and other drugs. Preventive Medicine 2000; 31(1):39–48.

10. Wolfson M, Forster JL, Claxton AJ, Murray DM. Adolescent smokers' provision of tobacco to other adolescents. American Journal of Public Health 1997; 87(4):649–651.

11. Forster J, Chen V, Blaine T, Perry C, Toomey T. Social exchange of cigarettes by youth. Tobacco Control 2003; 12(2):148–154.

12. Croghan E, Aveyard P, Griffin C, Cheng KK. The importance of social sources of cigarettes to school students. Tobacco Control 2003; 12(1):67–73.

13. Ma H, Unger JB, Chou C-P, *et al.* Risk factors for adolescent smoking in urban and rural China: Findings from the China seven cities study. Additive Behaviors 2008; 33(8):1081–1085.

14. Unger JB, Cruz T, Shakib S, *et al.* Exploring the cultural context of tobacco use: a transdisciplinary framework. Nicotine & Tobacco Research. 2003; 5(Supplement 1):S101–117.

15. Tu SP, Walsh M, Tseng B, Thompson B. Tobacco Use by Chinese American Men: An Exploratory Study of the Factors Associated with Cigarette Use and Smoking Cessation. Asian American and Pacific Islander Journal of Health 2000; 8(1):46–57.

16. Hu M, Rich ZC, Luo D, Xiao S. Cigarette sharing and gifting in rural China: a focus group study. Nicotine & Tobacco Research 2012; 14(3):361–367.

17. Rich ZC, Xiao S. Tobacco as a social currency: cigarette gifting and sharing in China. Nicotine & Tobacco Research 2012; 14(3):258–263.

18. Ding D, Hovell MF. Cigarettes, social reinforcement, and culture: a commentary on "Tobacco as a social currency: cigarette gifting and sharing in China". Nicotine & Tobacco Research. 2012; 14(3):255–257.

19. Pan Z. Socioeconomic predictors of smoking and smoking frequency in urban China: evidence of smoking as a social function. Health Promotion International 2004; 19(3):309–315.

20. O'Sullivan B, Chapman S. Eyes on the prize: transnational tobacco companies in China 1976–1997. Tobacco Control 2000; 9(3):292–302.

21. Chu A, Jiang N, Glantz SA. Transnational tobacco industry promotion of the cigarette gifting custom in China. Tobacco Control 2011; 20(4): e3–e3.

22. Bian Y. Guangxi and the allocation of urban jobs in china. The China Quarterly 1994; 140:971–999.

23. Yan Y. *The Flow of Gifts: Reciprocity and Social Networks in a Chinese Village.* 1st ed. Redwood City, CA: Stanford University Press; 1996.

24. Kohrman M. Depoliticizing Tobacco's Exceptionality: Male Sociality, Death and Memory-making among Chinese Cigarette Smokers. The China Journal 2007; 58: 85–109.

25. Hu TW, Lee AH, Mao Z. WHO Framework Convention on Tobacco Control in China: barriers, challenges and recommendations. Global Health Promotion 2013; 20(4):13–22.

26. Shan J. Cigarettes top New Year gift list: Poll. *China Daily.* February 5, 2010. http://www.chinadaily.com.cn/china/2010-02/05/content_9431234.htm (accessed March 11, 2014).

27. World Lung Foundation, Survey Indicates Fewer People in Beijing and Shanghai Intended to Give Cigarettes as Gifts after Seeing Mass Media Campaign. 2009; http://www.worldlungfoundation.org/ht/d/ReleaseDetails/i/6253. (accessed March 11, 2014).

28. WHO. WHO report on the global tobacco epidemic, 2008, The MPOWER package: WHO; 2008.

29. General Office of the CPC Central Committee and General Office of the State Council. Notice on Officials Shall Take the Lead in Making Public Places Smoke Free. http://news.xinhuanet.com/politics/2013-12/29/c_118753701.htm (accessed March 11, 2014).

Section III

Tobacco Taxation System and Its Reform Impact

Chapter 9

The Role of Taxation in Tobacco Control and Its Potential Economic Impact in China*

Teh-wei Hu, Zhengzhong Mao, Jian Shi and Wendong Chen

ABSTRACT

Objectives To identify key economic issues involved in raising the tobacco tax and to recommend possible options for tobacco tax reform in China.

Methods Estimated price elasticities of the demand for cigarettes, prevalence data and epidemiology are used to estimate the impact of a tobacco tax increase on cigarette consumption, government tax revenue, lives saved, employment and revenue loss in the cigarette industry and tobacco farming.

Results The recent Chinese tax adjustment, if passed along to the retail price, would reduce the number of smokers by 630 000 saving 210 000 lives, at a price elasticity of −0.15. A tax increase of 1 RMB (or US$0.13) per pack of cigarettes would increase the Chinese government's tax revenue by 129 billion RMB (US 17.2 billion), decrease consumption by 3.0 billion packs of cigarettes, reduce the number of smokers by 3.42 million and save 1.14 million lives.

Conclusion The empirical economic analysis and tax simulation results clearly indicate that increasing the tobacco tax in China is the most cost-effective instrument for tobacco control.

---

*Published in *Tobacco Control*, 2010; 19:58–64. doi: 10.1136/tc.2009.031799.

149

INTRODUCTION

China grows about one-third of the world's tobacco crop and consumes one-third of the world's cigarettes. The 2002 National Smoking Prevalence Survey estimated there to be about 300 million current smokers in China.[1]

The health and economic consequences of smoking are alarming. A recent estimate of mortality attributable to smoking in China is 673 000 deaths per year if limited to cancer, cardiovascular disease and respiratory disease.[2] And because diseases caused by smoking can take several decades to develop, China has yet to catch up to the high smoking-related mortality seen in the West.[3] Smoking attributable deaths in China are projected to rise to 2 million by the year 2020.[4]

The health burdens of smoking also can be measured in monetary cost, which includes medical treatment costs (direct costs) and loss of productivity from morbidity and mortality (indirect costs). A study that used the 1998 China National Health Services Survey estimated the smoking-attributable total costs of three major diseases — cancer, cardiovascular (CV) disease and respiratory disease — at 41.0 billion RMB (or US$5.0 billion, US$1 = 8.20RMB for the 2000 exchange rate) measured in 2000 value, or about 208 RMB (US $25.43) per smoker ($\geq$age 35).[5] The direct medical costs of smoking accounted for 3.1% of China's national health expenditures in 2000.[6]

To reduce this cost burden in the future, effective tobacco control programs and sustained efforts are needed to curb the tobacco epidemic and economic losses. One of the most important instruments a government can use in tobacco control is taxation. Worldwide experience has shown that raising the tax on cigarette sales is very effective in reducing consumption.[3]

The objectives of this paper are to identify key economic issues for evidence-based policy analysis, including the various aspects of tobacco taxation and to recommend possible options for tobacco tax reform in China.

The remainder of this paper is organised as follows. The next section reviews the tobacco economy in China. The third section provides a review of China's tax system with particular emphasis on the tobacco leaf tax and the cigarette tax. The fourth section describes tobacco price, affordability, consumption and demand analysis. The fifth section provides a simulation of the impact of tobacco tax income on China's economy and population health. Recommendations are included in the final section.

THE TOBACCO ECONOMY IN CHINA

The Chinese government plays an important role in the production of tobacco leaf and cigarettes through its national monopoly, the State Tobacco Administration (STMA) and the China National Tobacco Company (CNTC), one organisation with two names. The STMA sets overall government policy on tobacco, beginning with the allocation of tobacco production quotas among the provinces, the pricing of tobacco leaf, the setting of production quotas for cigarettes and the managing of international trade. The CNTC has the overall responsibility of setting national tobacco leaf production quotas for all provinces.

According to law, the CNTC is the only legitimate buyer of tobacco leaf in China. In 2005, China produced 2.435 million tons of tobacco leaf, about one-third of the world's production.[7] In the same year, the 1.363 million hectares planted with tobacco accounted for less than 1% of China's total agricultural cultivated land. The gross value of fluecured tobacco was 23.23 billion RMB, or 9.54 RMB per kg, contributing 1% to 2% to the Chinese agricultural economy.[7]

Currently, the Chinese central government allows the local government to keep 20% of tobacco leaf tax revenues. As a result, 24 of 31 provinces in China (about 4 million farm households or about 2% of all farmers) grow tobacco.[8] Almost all of these households also produce other crops. Of the 24 tobacco-producing provinces, Yunnan, Guizhou, Henan and Sichuan are the 4 most important in terms of growing tobacco and manufacturing cigarettes. According to the 2005 China Agricultural Statistics, the net return for tobacco leaf compared to its production cost was 22% for Yunnan and 18% for Henan, but only 1.25% for Guizhou and −4.98% for Sichuan.[9] These production costs included the imputed cost of farmers' own labour time, but not tobacco company subsidies to farmers, which explains how a negative return for Sichuan tobacco farmers is possible.

In 2007, China's state-owned tobacco monopoly produced 106.98 billion packs of cigarettes, generating a profit and tax of 388 billion RMB, about 7.56% of central government revenue.[10] The cigarette manufacturing industry employed about a half a million people, or about 0.06% of the total national employment. About 3.5 million persons were engaged in retail cigarette sales. However, very few persons were sole cigarette retailers and many worked on a part time basis; they comprised 0.6% of the total employed population in 2005.[8]

China entered the World Trade Organization (WTO) in 2001. With the WTO removing China's longstanding restrictions on tobacco imports and the numerous domestic companies within the state monopoly, the largest Chinese tobacco company cannot yet compete directly with the transnational tobacco companies. In recent years, foreign products have set their product price comparable to the most popular domestic brands, such as Hong Ta Shan brand or Zhong Hua brand. The CNTC anticipates that before the end of the decade, foreign products may reach 8% to 10% of the Chinese tobacco market.[7]

To compete with the transnational tobacco companies, CNTC has consolidated many regional companies to improve efficiency. One major consequence of these mergers is increased unemployment. The 92 small cigarette companies that were closed had about 59000 employees and 5500 retired employees. Chinese tobacco companies have begun addressing employment issues in light of this industry restructuring.

THE TAX SYSTEM AND TAX STRUCTURE IN CHINA

China has a central government tax and a local government tax. The central government collects a value-added tax (VAT), personal and enterprise income tax, specific excise tax and custom tax among others. The local government collects a business tax, special tobacco leaf tax and city construction/maintenance tax.

Even though the central government collects a large majority of the taxes in China, revenue from some of the collected taxes is shared with the local government. This revenue sharing provides financial incentives for the local government to collect taxes on behalf of the central government. China has two tobacco-related taxes: the tobacco leaf tax and the tobacco product (mainly cigarette) tax.

Before 2005, tobacco leaf was included under the agricultural tax, which was levied at 31% of the CNTC purchase price. The revenue from this special agricultural tax was collected and used for local government purposes. In 2006, the central government decided to eliminate all agricultural product taxes to relieve farmers' financial burdens. However, tobacco leaf was not included in the tax exemption. Instead, a special tobacco leaf tax was designed and the tax rate was reduced from 31% to 20%.[11] This local tobacco leaf tax serves as an incentive for local officials to encourage farmers to produce tobacco leaf above and beyond the CNTC quota, which leads to a surplus of tobacco leaf, which then becomes a source for underground private cigarette companies.

Before 1 May 2009, the cigarette tax rate in China consisted of two components: (1) a specific excise tax of 0.06 RMB per pack for all cigarettes and (2) an ad valorem tax of 45% for cigarettes with a producer price higher than or equal to 5 RMB per pack (class A cigarettes) and a 30% tax rate for cigarettes with a value less than 5 RMB per pack (class B cigarettes).

In late May 2009, the Chinese Ministry of Finance (MOF) and the State Administration of Taxation (SAT) announced an adjustment to the cigarette product tax. While the specific excise tax of 0.06 RMB per pack remained unchanged, the ad valorem tax structure was changed as follows: (1) an ad valorem tax of 56% is levied on cigarettes with a producer price higher than or equal to 7 RMB per pack (class A cigarettes) and a 36% tax on cigarettes with a value less than 7 RMB per pack (class B cigarettes), and (2) an additional 5% tax is applied to the whole price, which includes the new increases in the producer price tax.

Table 1 provides a comparison of the Chinese tobacco tax structure before and after May 2009. The government indicated that the purpose of the new adjustment is to increase government revenue from cigarette products. It requires the CNTC to absorb all of the additional tax from its profits, not

Table 1:   Comparison of Chinese Tobacco Excise Tax Structure Before and After 1 May 2009

	Before 1 May 2009	After 1 May 2009
Specific excise tax per pack	0.06 RMB	0.06 RMB
Ad valorem tax		
Price per pack	≥5RMB 45%	≥7RMB 56%
Price per pack	<5 RMB 30%	<7RMB 36%
Wholesale price tax*	0%	5%

*Wholesale price includes the amount of ad valorem tax.

allowing the new tax adjustment to be passed along to the retail level. Thus, the same cigarette tax rate is maintained at the retail level in China.

Under the tax structure in effect before May 2009, the Chinese government claimed that China's cigarette tax was about 65% at the producer price level.[6] Using the $t/(t+1)$ equation and a 65% tax rate (t) at the producer price level, the cigarette tax rate in China would be about 40% at the retail price level. International practice calculates the cigarette tax at a retail price level to reflect consumers' financial outlay in buying cigarettes.

If the Chinese government were to pass along the additional producer/wholesale tax increase to the retail price, the weighted tax rate at the producer price level would be an additional 11.7 percentage points, assuming the recent mark-up between producer price and wholesale price and the weighted sales value distribution among the two classes of cigarettes.[12] Thus, the adjusted tax rate at the producer price level would be 76.7% (65% + 11.7%), and the new retail price tax rate would become 43.4% (76.7%/(1 + 76.7%)), an increase of 3.4 percentage points.[12] More than 50 countries around the world have higher retail cigarette tax rates than these effective tax rates in China.[13]

To maintain sufficient local government revenue, the central government transfers 25% of the VAT revenue to the local government. Furthermore, the central government also transfers 40% of enterprises' income tax revenues to the local government. This form of tax revenue sharing provides an incentive to local government to protect its local tobacco industry by controlling tobacco leaf production, marketing and pricing. The national tobacco monopoly industry becomes many localised monopolies.

One reason the Chinese government pays significant attention to the tobacco industry is the latter's contribution to the central government's collected revenues. The CNTC is a government-owned monopoly that combines its profit and tax revenue as revenues. In 1995, the tobacco industry contributed about 11.4% of total central government revenue; its contribution declined to 7.56% in 2007. The recent fall in the proportion of the tobacco tax to total tax is due to higher tax revenues from China's burgeoning export market rather than any reduction in tobacco production or manufacturing of tobacco products. However, even though its relative share in government revenue has been declining, the tobacco industry is still a very important source of revenue for the central government in China.

PRICE, AFFORDABILITY, CONSUMPTION AND DEMAND ANALYSIS

The price of cigarettes is a key variable when considering the use of taxation as an instrument for tobacco control. In 1990, the nominal retail price per pack of cigarettes in China was 1.088 RMB; it then increased gradually to 6.641 RMB in 2007, as shown in Table 2. According to the consumer price index (CPI), using 1990 as 100, the overall price of cigarettes increased 2.28 times during that period; using the CPI to deflate the nominal cigarette price, the per pack price in 2007 measured at the 1990 price level, was 2.91 RMB per pack.

To address the affordability of cigarettes, one can divide per capita disposable income by the price per pack of cigarettes each year. Then, using

Table 2:   Cigarette Prices, Affordability Index and Consumption (1990–2007)

Year	Nominal Retail Price (RMB/ Pack)	Consumer Price Index (1990 = 100)	Real Retail Cigarette Price (1990 = 100) (RMB/ Pack)	Proxy Disposable Income Per Capita (RMB)	Affordability Index	Per Capita Consumption (Packs/Year)
1990	1.088	100.0	1.088	1637	1.000	65.97
1991	1.207	103.4	1.168	1884	1.038	67.64
1992	1.328	110.0	1.207	2298	1.150	66.15
1993	1.421	126.2	1.126	2975	1.391	68.99
1994	1.564	156.6	0.998	4014	1.706	68.29
1995	1.736	183.4	0.946	4938	1.890	70.17
1996	1.944	198.6	0.979	5731	1.959	67.77
1997	2.177	204.2	1.066	6314	1.928	68.54
1998	2.316	202.5	1.144	6654	1.910	65.82
1999	2.464	199.7	1.234	7034	1.897	64.50
2000	2.585	200.5	1.289	7732	1.988	60.95
2001	2.793	201.9	1.383	8467	2.015	64.60
2002	3.086	200.3	1.541	9271	1.997	68.09
2003	3.420	202.7	1.687	10460	2.033	69.57
2004	3.899	210.6	1.851	12277	2.093	72.09
2005	4.522	214.4	2.109	14128	2.076	71.81
2006	5.384	217.6	2.474	16214	2.328	77.41
2007	6.641	228.0	2.913	19033	2.340	80.96

Sources: China's Statistics Yearbook (1989–2008), China National Bureau of Statistics, Beijing, China; China Tobacco Statistics Yearbook (1989–2008), China National Tobacco Company, Beijing, China.

the base year (1990) ratio as a denominator for each subsequent year (eg, 1991, 1992 and so on), one can derive an affordability index, a measure of price relative to income. With rapid economic growth in China between 1990 and 2007, the nominal proxy index of the per capita disposable income increased from 1637 RMB in 1990 to 19 033 RMB in 2007, about 11.63 times. This increase in disposable income indicates that Chinese consumers' income increased much faster than the price of cigarettes, by almost 2.34 times between 1990 and 2007. Thus, cigarettes in China became more than twice as affordable between 1990 and 2007. As shown in Table 2, given that the relatively low increase in the real price has made cigarettes more affordable over time, per capita cigarette consumption has been increasing since 2000.

Demand Analysis and Price Elasticity

Determining the impact of taxation on cigarette consumption and subsequently on government revenue requires an analysis of the relation between price and consumption of cigarettes. The relationship can be expressed in quantitative measures. Price elasticity is particularly important since it measures the effect on consumption of a change in price.

Past empirical estimated price elasticities range widely from −0.007 to −0.84,[14−21] due mainly to variations in the data sets (time series vs cross section; aggregate vs individual observations), model specification and estimated methods. However, they can be grouped into three categories based on their magnitudes. (1) The high-end price elasticities, around −0.80, were obtained from two time series studies.[14,15] Although international literature often cites −0.80 as the price elasticity among developing countries, it seems unlikely that Chinese smokers would have such a high response to price change in the short term; this could be a long-term price elasticity.[16] (2) The middle range of elasticities, from −0.50 to −0.60, represents almost half of all estimated results and is cited mostly in the literature from middle-income or high-income countries.[17−19] (3) The low-end price elasticities, from −0.007 to −0.154, are from the most recent Chinese studies and based on much larger nationally representative data sources.[20,21] One possible explanation for the low price elasticity in China is the availability of cigarettes with a wide range of prices, from 2.0 RMB (US$0.15) to 200 RMB (US $24.4) per pack, suggesting that smokers can easily switch to lower priced brands without quitting. Furthermore, due to the rapid income growth in the Chinese economy, cigarettes have become much more affordable, thus reducing the price effect.

Since the magnitude of price elasticity is one of the most important parameters used to simulate the impact of a cigarette tax on cigarette consumption, government revenue, population health and the overall economy, we will use two different price elasticities of −0.15 and −0.50 for a short-term tax impact sensitivity analysis. The estimated elasticity of −0.15 of the demand for cigarettes consists of two components: the probability of being a smoker, that is, the participation elasticity was −0.06 and the price elasticity of the demand for the amount of cigarettes conditional on being a smoker was −0.09.[21] Thus, approximately 40% of the decline in cigarette consumption in China was from quitting (or not initiating) smoking, and 60% of the decline was from current smokers reducing their consumption.

SIMULATION OF THE IMPACT OF SPECIFIC EXCISE TAX INCREASES

Impact on Cigarette Consumption, Government Tax Revenue and Health

Two different potential tax increases are used for the simulation: (1) the new 43.4% tax rate that would result from the May 2009 tax adjustment structure if the producer tax adjustment was passed on to the retail level by the Chinese government and (2) an increase of 1 RMB per pack specific excise tax (currently less than 0.06 RMB per pack), above and beyond the recent tax adjustment, a more administratively effective strategy with a potentially larger impact on tobacco control. The results discussed below are shown in Table 3.

(1) China sold 106.98 billion packs of cigarettes in 2007. Under the new adjusted tax rate of 43.4%, the 2007 retail price of 6.64 RMB per pack would have increased to 6.87 RMB (or 0.23 RMB), and 0.54 billion fewer packs would have been sold at −0.15 price elasticity and 1.82 billion fewer packs sold at −0.50 price elasticity. An additional 1 RMB excise tax would result in a reduction in sales, respectively, of 3.0 billion packs and 9.96 billion packs.

Under a price elasticity of −0.15 and a smoking participation elasticity of −0.06, the prevalence rate of smoking would be reduced from 31% to 30.8% or from 308 million smokers to 307.37 million smokers, a reduction of

Table 3: The Impact of Cigarette Tax Increases on Tobacco-Attributable Mortality and Government Tax Revenue Using Different Price Elasticities

	2007 Levels	Recent Tax Adjustment	Increase in Specific Excise Tax of Additional 1 RMB
Increase in cigarette tax per pack (RMB)			
Cigarette retail price (RMB/pack)	*6.64*	6.87	7.87
Producer price	*3.98*	3.98	3.98
Tax per pack	*2.66*	2.89	3.89
Total tax as % of retail price	40%	43.4%	50.6%
Reduction in cigarette consumption (billion packs)			
0.15*		0.54	3.00
0.50*		1.82	9.90
Reduction in number of smokers (millions)			
Price elasticities[†]			
0.15		0.63	3.42
0.50		2.09	11.41
Number of lives saved (millions)[‡]			
0.15		0.21	1.14
0.50		0.70	3.80
Prevalence of adult (aged 15+) current smokers (millions)	31%		
0.15		30.8%	30.13%
0.50		30.5%	28.13%
Total number of current smokers (millions)	308.0		
0.15		307.37	304.6
0.50		305.91	296.6
Additional total tax revenues (billions RMB)			
0.15		22.58	129.4
0.50		19.63	101.8
Total annual cigarette tax revenue (in US$)[§]			
0.15		3.01	17.25
0.50		2.62	13.57

*Price elasticity.
[†]Smoking participation elasticity = 40% of the total price elasticity; smoking intensity elasticity = 60% of the total price elasticity.
[‡]Assuming one-third reduction in smokers.[13]
[§]US$1 = 7.5 RMB for the 2007 exchange rate.

640,000 smokers with the passing of the latest tax adjustment to the retail level. Using the estimated epidemiology analysis reported by the *Tobacco Atlas* that indicates one-third of smokers (a high estimate could be half of all smokers) will die from tobacco-related illness,[13] a 3.4% tax increase would mean 210,000 lives could be saved. At the same time, government revenue would increase by an additional 22.58 billion RMB (US $3.01 billion at US$1 = 7.5 RMB, 2007 exchange rate).

At a price elasticity of −0.50 (i.e., smoking participation elasticity at −0.20, or 40% of −0.50) with a 3.4% tax increase, the prevalence rate of smoking would be reduced further from 31% to 30.5%, a reduction of 2.09 million smokers. If one-third of smokers will die prematurely, about 700 000 lives could be saved. Total government revenue could be increased by 19.63 billion RMB (US $2.62 billion).

(2) With an additional 1 RMB per pack increase, or at a retail price of 7.87 RMB per pack under a total price elasticity of −0.15, smoking participation elasticity would be −0.06 and the prevalence rate of smoking would be reduced from 31% to 30.13%, a reduction of 3.42 million smokers. Assuming one-third of smokers will die from tobacco-related illness,[13] a 1.00 RMB specific excise tax increase would mean 1.14 million lives could be saved. At the same time, the total government cigarette tax revenue would increase by 129.4 billion (or US$17.25 billion).

This same methodology also was used to estimate the impact of adding an additional 1 RMB excise tax per pack of cigarettes on cigarette consumption, health and government revenue assuming a total price elasticity of −0.50 (i.e., smoking participation elasticity at −0.20). In this scenario, the prevalence rate of smoking would be reduced further from 31% to 28.13%, a reduction of 11.41 million smokers. Again assuming one-third of smokers will die from tobacco-related illness, an additional 1.00 RMB specific excise tax would mean 3.80 million lives could be saved. The total government cigarette tax revenue would increase by 101.8 billion RMB (US$13.57 billion).

Not included in Table 3 are the potential cost savings in medical services and increased productivity resulting from the decreased number of smokers attributable to the increase in the tobacco tax. Under the cost of smoking analysis,[4] per smoker medical costs were about 200 RMB (US$26.67). If the Chinese government decides to pass along the additional 3.4% tax to smokers, 630 000 fewer smokers would result in savings of 126 million

RMB (US$168 million) in medical costs when the price elasticity is −0.15, or 418 million RMB (US55.7 million) when the price elasticity is −0.50. If the specific excise tax is raised an additional 1 RMB per pack, the resultant 3.42 million fewer smokers would result in savings of 684 million RMB (US$92.2 million) in medical costs when the price elasticity is −0.15 and 2.28 billion RMB (US$0.30 billion) if the price elasticity is −0.50.

The indirect cost of smoking in China can be estimated using the human capital approach, which is one method for evaluating the monetary value of life years lost, based on average forgone earnings of an individual as a loss of productivity to society.[5] The average per person loss of productivity due to premature death would be 2935 RMB measured at the 2000 present value. With 1.14 million lives saved with an increase of 1 RMB per pack in the excise tax, productivity would increase by 3.34 billion RMB (US$0.45 billion) at a price elasticity of −0.15. When the price elasticity is increased to −0.50, the number of lives saved would be 3.80 million and 10.27 billion (US$1.37 billion) would be generated for the Chinese economy.

In summary, these simulation estimates indicate that a cigarette tax increase in China would save lives, reduce medical care costs and increase productivity.

Impact of Cigarette Tax Increases on the Cigarette Industry and Tobacco Farming

The Chinese government's concerns that an increase in cigarette taxes will reduce cigarette consumption could have a minor effect on the cigarette industry, given the population expansion in China even if per capita consumption decreases. The potential short-term impacts of a tax increase can be simulated. When an additional tax is levied on cigarettes, the immediate impact is a reduction in sales, which will lead to a reduction in revenue as well as employment in the cigarette industry. Under the recent tax adjustment scenario, as shown in Table 4, the reduction of cigarette consumption could be between 0.54 billion and 1.82 billion packs, depending on a price elasticity of −0.15 or −0.50. The industry sales revenue loss (based on 3.98 RMB per pack 2007 producer price as shown in Table 3) would be between 2.08 billion RMB and 6.86 billion RMB. Its employment loss would be very minimal, between 279 and 936 persons. If an additional 1 RMB excise tax were imposed, the industry total sales revenue loss would be 11.94 billion RMB. Excluding the

Table 4: The Impact of Cigarette Tax Increases on the Cigarette Industry and Tobacco Farming Using Different Price Elasticities

	Recent Tax Adjustment	Increase in Specific Excise Tax of Additional 1 RMB
Impact on cigarette industry		
Reduction in cigarette consumption (billion packs)		
0.15*	0.54	3.0
0.50*	1.82	9.90
Total sales revenue loss (billion RMB)[†]		
0.15	2.08	11.94
0.50	6.86	39.40
Industry net revenue loss (billion RMB)[‡]		
0.15	1.17	6.71
0.50	3.85	22.15
Industry employment loss (number of employees)		
0.15	279	1606
0.50	936	5382
Impact on tobacco farming		
Reduction in tobacco leaf (in tons)[§]		
0.15	4397	25271
0.50	14734	84677
Reduction in land use (in hectares)[¶]		
0.15	2429	13960
0.50	8139	44778
Reduction in farmers' revenue (in millions RMB)**		
0.15	44	253
0.50	147	847
Reduction in local government tax (in millions RMB)[††]		
0.15	8.7	50
0.50	29.4	169

Notes:
*Price elasticity.
[†]Total sales revenue loss is the producer price 3.98 RMB (6.64–2.66) RMB per pack multiplied by the reduction in consumption.
[‡]Figures obtained from Table 2.
[§]0.041 tons of tobacco leaf produce 1 case of cigarettes (50 000 cigarettes).[6]
[¶]Average productivity is 1.81 tons per hectare.
**Average government purchase price was 500 RMB per 50 kg, 10 000 RMB per ton (1 ton = 1000 kg).
[††]20% special tobacco leaf tax.

production costs and tax contribution to the government, the net loss to the industry would be 6.71 billion RMB in sales revenue, only 0.52% (6.71/129.4) of the total additional revenue the government would gain from the increased tax.[6] The average profit of the cigarette manufacturing industry is 10.3% of total revenue.[6] Thus, the loss of profit would be 691 million RMB. Compared to the gain in government revenue of 129.4 billion RMB, the net loss to the cigarette industry would be very small.

Under the assumption of a price elasticity of −0.50, with an increase of additional 1 RMB per pack in excise tax, the reduction in cigarette sales would be 9.90 billion packs. The average producer cigarette price was 3.98 RMB; thus, the total gross sales revenue loss would be 39.4 billion RMB, as shown in Table 4. The net industry loss would be 22.15 billion, and the net profit loss would be 2.28 billion RMB.

If we consider employment as a linear function of production volume, then a 1.6% loss of sales in the cigarette industry under a price elasticity of −0.15, as shown in Table 4, would result in a drop in employment rates by the same percentage, or about 1606 employees. Under a price elasticity of −0.50, with a 5.3% loss of sales, the employment loss would be 5382 employees. Compared to the loss of 59 000 employees due to company merging, the employment loss from an increase in taxes would be minimal.

An increase in tax and reduction in cigarette consumption may provide further impetus to improve the efficiency of cigarette production. The effect of the reduction in cigarette consumption could lead the cigarette manufacturing industry to diversify into other products. Furthermore, the amount of money that smokers save from reduced cigarette consumption could be spent on food or household goods. Therefore, the net effect on employment could be even smaller than estimated. Studies in the USA, UK and Indonesia[22–24] using their national input/output industry tables, showed that a cigarette tax increase led to a gain in income and employment in other sectors greater than the decline in the true tobacco sector.

Considering the loss of revenue for the cigarette industry and income for industry employees, the government could grant subsidies to the cigarette industry and their employees to retrain workers displaced by higher tobacco taxes and transfer them to other manufacturing industries as well as provide alternative production opportunities, the same steps taken by the Chinese tobacco industry during its restructuring.

One of the major concerns of the Chinese government with respect to raising the tobacco tax is its potential negative economic impact on tobacco farmers' livelihood. To estimate the possible economic impact of a tobacco tax increase on tobacco farming, one can first examine the demand and supply relationship between a reduction in the demand for cigarettes and the magnitude of a cigarette price increase (i.e., due to a tax increase). Given the predicted reduction in the demand for cigarettes, one can use a simple linear production relationship between the input requirement (tobacco leaf) and a produced pack of cigarettes. One can further simulate the monetary value lost from not producing tobacco leaf by multiplying the average government purchase price by the amount of tobacco leaf not sold in the market.

Chinese tobacco industry statistics indicate that 0.041 ton of tobacco leaf is required to produce 1 case (or 50 000 pieces) of cigarettes.[25] Thus, an additional 3.4% tax increase would lead to a reduction in the need for 4.397 tons of tobacco leaf. An additional 1 RMB tax increase would lead to a reduction in the need for 25 271 tons of tobacco leaf, as shown in Table 4. Since the impact of the recent tax adjustment on tobacco farming is very small as shown in Table 4, only simulation results for a 1 RMB tax increase will be discussed here. The productivity relationship between tobacco leaf and hectares is 1.81 tons per hectare.[25] Thus an additional 1 RMB tax increase would reduce land use for tobacco farming by about 13 960 hectares, about 2% of total land use. The reduction in tobacco leaf sales would reduce tobacco farmers' income. The government purchase price for the middlegrade tobacco leaf ranged from 755 RMB per 50 kg for tobacco leaf from Yunnan and Guizhou provinces to 500 RMB (or top 505 RMB) for leaf from Northern Chinese provinces.[7] A 500 RMB price was picked for the analysis so that this purchase price could also be used to simulate the tax impact at the national level. The estimated revenue loss to farmers would be 253 million RMB from an additional 1 RMB per pack tax increase. Compared to the total national value of tobacco leaf sales, this revenue loss would be about 2.0% of total tobacco revenue. Considering the cost of producing tobacco leaf, the reduction in local government revenue would be 50 million RMB nationally. In 2007, the local government in China collected 4.646 billion RMB in local tax; the reduction of 50 million RMB represents a loss of 0.30% of total revenue. These losses could be replenished by the gain of 129.4 billion RMB in tax revenue by the central government.

In summary, an additional 1 RMB tax increase on cigarettes would not have a serious effect on either tobacco farmers' income or local government tax revenue. In fact, the alternative use of this tobacco land could be even more beneficial, based on farm household survey results on costs and returns on tobacco leaf production.[26] As shown in Table 4, under the assumption of a price elasticity of −0.50, a similar simulation can be estimated for an additional 1 RMB specific excise tax increase per pack of cigarettes. Again, farmers would use the land to produce other profitable crops. The central government would generate an additional 101.8 billion RMB, six times the loss of local government revenue. These local government revenue losses could be easily compensated for by the financial gain of the central government.

Finally, one major concern raised by the Chinese government is the regressivity of a tobacco tax increase. Low-income smokers in China pay less per pack and smoke fewer cigarettes than highincome smokers. Furthermore, low-income smokers are more price responsive than high-income smokers. Therefore, the savings from tobacco expenditures for low-income smokers could be used for other household necessities, such as food, clothing and housing, potentially leading to an improvement in their general standard of living.

RECOMMENDATIONS

The Chinese government claims that its cigarette tax rate is about 65% of the producer price, which is about 40% of the retail price. Even if the recent tax adjustment is passed along to the retail level, it is only 43.4% of the retail price. Thus, China has room to raise the tax on cigarettes. The empirical economic analysis and tax simulation results presented in this paper clearly support the policy position that increasing the tobacco tax in China is a most cost-effective instrument for tobacco control. We therefore suggest the following recommendations.

Increase the Cigarette Tax

To achieve the goal of tobacco control, the Chinese government should first pass along its recent tobacco tax increase from the producer/wholesale price to the retail price and then significantly increase the specific excise tax on cigarettes, which is currently 0.06 RMB per pack by at least an additional 1 RMB per pack. Raising the specific excise tax would narrow the dispersion between low-end and higher-end brand prices and be an effective tax instrument for tobacco control. In addition, the government should simplify the current two-tier ad valorem tax into one single rate to prevent producers from arbitrarily adjusting the brand price to pay a lower tax rate. To maintain the effectiveness of tobacco control, the specific excise tax should be adjusted by the annual inflation rate. In the long run, China should consider increasing the overall tax rate beyond 60%, a figure common in many other countries.

Remove the Tobacco Leaf Tax

The Chinese government should consider removing the special tobacco leaf tax. Because this is a recently established (2006) tax category, the Chinese government may be reluctant to remove the tax right away because of the immediate potential negative fiscal impact on some local economic development projects. However, the current pervasive incentive for local government to encourage farmers to plant tobacco leaf leads to surplus tobacco leaf, one of the major sources of counterfeit (tobacco) cigarettes. Instead, the central government could increase the cigarette tax and then transfer part of the additional cigarette tax revenue to local government to compensate for its losses resulting from the elimination of the special tobacco leaf tax. At the same time, this strategy would free tobacco farmers to plant any crop they desire. Some of the additional cigarette tax revenue could be used by the Chinese government to subsidise tobacco farmers wishing to substitute other crops for tobacco leaf. Chinese Ministry of Agricultural and international organisations such as Food and Agricultural Organisation (FAO) should provide technical assistance for tobacco farmers on crop substitution.

What this paper adds

- This paper provides a concrete recommendation for tobacco tax policy.
- It also provides comprehensive estimates of the impact of a tobacco tax increase on the Chinese economy.

Reform Revenue Sharing Between the Central and Local Government

The Chinese government should consider removing the tobacco tax revenue sharing between the central government and the local government and use the existing central government revenue transfer mechanism between the central government and local government to support local fiscal needs. In the future, the contributions of the cigarette industry to government revenue may become smaller, given the increasing importance of multinational tobacco companies in the Chinese tobacco market. The role of the Chinese central government should be to pursue a more aggressive tobacco control strategy, consistent with the World Health organization Framework Convention on Tobacco Control (WHO FCTC) provision to increase the tobacco tax, without worrying about tobacco control barriers at the provincial level.

Earmark the Additional Tax Revenue

The Chinese government should consider using the additional cigarette tax revenue for tobacco control activities, such as media antismoking campaigns, enforcement of non-smoking legislation and coverage of healthcare expenses for the lowincome population. Many other countries, such as the USA, Thailand, Australia, the UK and others have earmarked part of their cigarette tax revenues for health insurance and health promotion programs. The combined price and non-price tobacco control campaigns will maximise China's efforts towards tobacco regulation.

ACKNOWLEDGEMENTS

The authors are grateful for the suggestions and comments provided by Dr Tom Frieden, former New York Health Commissioner, Dr Kelly Henning and Dr Julie Myers of the Bloomberg Initiative to Reduce Tobacco Use, Dr Frank Chaloupka, Dr Hana Ross, Dr Emil Sunley and Dr Judith Mackay. We would like to thank Dr Hai-Yen Sung of the University of California, San Francisco, who provided simulation analyses for the demand model. This paper is condensed from a report prepared for the Bloomberg Initiative to Reduce Tobacco Use — Tobacco Taxation and its Potential Impact in China (Teh-wei Hu, Zhengzhong Mao, Jian Shin, Wendong Chen), December

2008. The authors remain responsible for the contents of the paper, and the views expressed herein do not represent those of the authors' affiliations.

Contributors T-wH designed the study and prepared the text. ZM analysed the data and provided interpretations, while WC and JS collected data and reviewed findings.

Funding US National Institutes of Health, Fogarty International Center (R01-TW05938) and the International Union Against Tuberculosis and Lung Disease.

Competing Interests None.

Provenance and Peer Review Not commissioned; externally peer reviewed.

REFERENCES

1. China Ministry of Health. *China smoking and health report 2006.* Beijing: Ministry of Health, 2006.
2. Gu D, Kelly T, Wu X, *et al.* Mortality attributable to smoking in China. *N Engl J Med* 2009;**360**:150–9.
3. World Bank. *Curbing the epidemic: government and the economics of tobacco control.* Washington, DC: World Bank, 1999.
4. Liu BQ, Peto R, Chen ZM, *et al.* Emerging tobacco hazards in China: 1. Retrospective proportional mortality study of one million deaths. *BMB* 1998;**317**:1411–22.
5. Sung HY, Wang L, Jin S, *et al.* Economic burden of smoking in China, 2000. *Tob Control* 2006;**15**:5–11.
6. China National Institute of Health Economics. *China national health expenditure report.* Beijing, China: Chinese Ministry of Health, 2006.
7. Liu TN, Xiong B. Tobacco economy and tobacco control. Beijing, China: Economic Science Press, 2004.
8. Tao M. *China tobacco industry under monopoly system: theory, problems, and system reform [in Chinese].* Shanghai (China): Xiulin (Academic) Press, 2005.
9. National Development and Reform Commission. *Collection of Cost and Return Survey for all national agricultural products.* Beijing, China: National Bureau of Statistics, 2005.
10. China National Bureau of Statistics. *China statistical yearbook.* Beijing, China: National Bureau of Statistics, 2008.
11. State Council. People's Republic of China Temporary Law on Tobacco Leaf Tax. 2006, 8 April.
12. Hu T, Mao Z, Shi J. Recent tobacco tax rate adjustment and its potential impact on tobacco control in China. *A paper presented at the International Health Economics Conference,* Beijing, July 12, 2009.

13. Shafey O, Eriksen M, Ross H, *et al. The tobacco atlas.* 3rd edn. Atlanta (Georgia, USA): American Cancer Society, 2009.

14. Mao ZZ, Jiang JL. Demand for cigarette and pricing policy (in Chinese). *Chinese Health Economics* 1997;**16**:50–2.

15. Bai Y, Zhang Z. Aggregate cigarette demand and regional differences in China. *Applied Economics* 2005;**37**:2523–28.

16. Chaloupka FJ, Warner KE. The economics of smoking. In Culyer AJ, Newhouse JP, eds. *Handbook of health economics.* Amsterdam: Elsevier, 2000: 1539–1627.

17. Hu TW, Mao Z. Effects of cigarette tax on cigarette consumption and the Chinese economy. *Tob Control* 2002;**11**:105–8.

18. Mao Z, Hu TW, Yang GH. New estimate of the demand for cigarettes in China (in Chinese). *Chinese J Health Econ* 2005;**24**:45–7.

19. Mao Z, Yang GH, Ma H. Adults' demand for cigarettes and its determinants in China (in Chinese). *Soft Science of Health* 2003;**17**:19–23.

20. Lance P, Akin J, Dow W, *et al.* Is cigarette smoking in poorer nations highly sensitive to price? Evidence from Russia and China. *J Health Econ* 2004;**23**:173–89.

21. Mao Z, Hu TW, Yang GH. Price elasticities and impact of tobacco tax among various income groups (in Chinese). *Chinese Journal of Evidence-Based Medicine* 2005;**5**:291–5.

22. Warner KE, Fulton GA, Nicholas P, *et al.* Employment implications of declining tobacco product sales for the regional economics of the United States. *JAMA* 1996;**275**:1241–6.

23. Buck D, Godfrey C, Raw M, *et al. Society for the study of addiction and centre for health economics.* York (England): University of York, 1995.

24. Alisan A, Wigonu I. The impact of higher cigarette tax to the Indonesian economy. Presentation at the South East Asian Tobacco Control Alliance Workshop, Bangkok, Nov. 27–28, 2007.

25. Wang S, Li B. Analysis and estimate of the situation of China's tobacco sector. *Sino World Tobacco* 2000;**47**:6–11.

26. Hu T, Mao Z, Jiang H, *et al.* The role of government in tobacco leaf production in China: National and local interventions. *Int J Public Policy* 2007;**2**:235–48.

Chapter 10

Recent Tobacco Tax Rate Adjustment and Its Potential Impact on Tobacco Control in China*

Teh-wei Hu, Zhengzhong Mao and Jian Shi

ABSTRACT

Objectives To compare the new tobacco tax structure effective from May 2009 with the tax structure before May 2009 and to analyse its potential impact.

Methods Published government statistics and estimated price elasticities of the demand for cigarettes are used to estimate the impact of the new tax rate adjustment on cigarette consumption and population health.

Results The new adjustment increased the tax rate by 11.7% points at the producer price level. Converting this 11.7% point increase to the retail price level would mean an increase of 3.4% points in the retail price tax rate. Thus, China's new cigarette tax rate at the retail level would be 43.4% instead of the previous 40%.

Conclusions The primary motivation for the recent Chinese government tobacco tax adjustment is to raise additional government revenue. Because the additional ad valorem tax has not yet been transferred to smokers, there is no public health benefit. It is hoped that the Chinese government will pass along these taxes to the retail price level, which would result in between 640 000 and two million smokers quitting smoking and between 210 000 and 700 000 quitters avoiding smoking-related premature death.

---

*Published in *Tobacco Control*, 2010; 19:80–82. doi: 10.1136/tc.2009.032631.

INTRODUCTION

In late May 2009; the Chinese Ministry of Finance and the State Administration of Taxation issued Taxation Document No. 84. 'The Notice Regarding Adjustment to Tobacco Product Excise Tax Policy',[1] effective from 1 May 2009. The adjustment is as follows:

1. The ad valorem tax for Class A cigarettes increases from 45% to 56%.
2. The ad valorem tax for Class B cigarettes increases from 30% to 36%.
3. All adjustments are levied on the producer price. Class A cigarettes are those costing 7 RMB ($US1.03, $US = 6.80 RMB at 2009 exchange rate) per pack or higher at the producer level, and Class cigarettes cost less than 7 RMB per pack. Before 1 May 2009 5 RMB ($0.74) was the class benchmark.
4. An additional 5% tax is applied to the wholesale price, after adding the new increases in the ad valorem tax.

According to the document, the purpose of this adjustment is to increase government revenue from cigarette products and also to improve the cigarette tax structure.

The producers and wholesale prices of various cigarette brands are jointly determined by the China National Tobacco Company (CNTC) and the State Pricing Bureau within the National Development and Reform Commission, according to Article 17, Peoples' Republic of China Tobacco Monopoly Act. The wholesale price for Chinese cigarettes is usually set by the State Taxation Monopoly Administration at 40% above the producer price for Class A cigarettes and 30% above the producer price for Class cigarettes.[2] Imposing a 5% additional tax on the wholesale price for Class A brands implies that the tax base for the wholesale price (P_w) is 2.184 P_p (Pp $(1+56\%)(1+40\%)$), where P_p is the producer price. Likewise, the tax base for the wholesale price (P_w) for Class B cigarettes is 1.768 P_p ($P_p(1+36\%)(1+30\%)$). The 5% wholesale tax increase converted into the producer price tax rate is 10.9% (2.184 × 5%) for Class A cigarettes and 8.8% (1.768 × 5%) for Class B cigarettes. Therefore, the new combined producer price tax rate and wholesale price tax rate at the producer price level is 66.9% (56% + 10.9%) for Class A brands and 44.8% (36% + 8.8%) for Class B brands. In other words, the new ad valorem tax rate is 21.9% higher (66.9%–45%) for Class A cigarettes and 14.8% higher (44.8%–30%) for Class B cigarettes than under the old tax structure.

The Class B brands, which cost between 5 RMB ($0.74) and 7 RMB ($1.03) per pack at the producer level, were taxed at 45% under the old tax structure and are now taxed at 36% under the new tax structure. However, if one includes the new 5% tax increase on the wholesale price, the resultant 44.8% (36% + 8.8%) tax rate is less than 0.2% point, but very close to the previous 45% level. This finding implies that there may not be a tax rate increase for brands costing between 5 RMB and 7 RMB per pack at the producer level.

The taxation document does not mention whether this tax adjustment is related to the Chinese government's 2005 ratification of the WHO Framework Convention on Tobacco Control (FCTC), and specifically to its compliance with Article VI on raising tobacco tax rates. On the other hand, it is possible that this adjustment will have positive effects on tobacco control in China if these additional taxes are shifted to the retail price. Raising the tobacco tax is considered one of the most effective policy instruments for tobacco control.

With a slowdown of the Chinese economy in early 2009, the Chinese government was seeking additional tax revenue to stimulate the economy. Because the Chinese National Tobacco Company (CNTC) is a government monopoly agency, the government can require the CNTC to transfer any additional profit to the government as fiscal revenue. We believe that this new tobacco tax adjustment was designed to serve as a formal basis for the funds to be transferred as well as a prelude for the central government to reform its tobacco tax structure. The intent of this adjustment is to make higher priced cigarettes (Class A) more expensive relative to lower priced cigarettes (Class B). The Taxation Document No. 84 specified that the additional taxes will be absorbed by the CNTC and not transferred to the retail price. There are two possible reasons for this requirement: political and economic. First is the political reason, that is, the Chinese government does not want to disturb smokers, especially the low-income smokers experiencing additional economic stress under the sluggish economy. Second is the economic reason — that is, the central government understands that CNTC has a comfortable profit margin and could absorb this additional tax burden, thereby potentially resulting in the CNTC becoming more efficient to maintain its net profit.

The purpose of this note is (1) to compare the new tax structure with the previous tax structure, which was implemented in 2001, and (2) to analyse the potential impact of the new tax structure on the Chinese government's tax revenue as well as its short-term and long-term impacts on cigarette consumption.

COMPARISON OF THE NEW TAX STRUCTURE WITH THE OLD TAX STRUCTURE

Table 1 compares the structure of the Chinese tobacco tax before and after 1 May 2009.[3] The specific excise tax (0.06 RMB per pack) remained the same. Under the new tax structure, the ad valorem tax increased from 45% to 56%, an 11% point increase for cigarettes with a producer price of 7 RMB per pack or higher. For brands priced at least 5 RMB but less than 7 RMB, the new tax rate is actually 9% points less than under the old tax structure. For brands costing less than 5 RMB, the tax rate increased 6% points. In addition, a new across-the-board 5% point tax is based on the wholesale price, which includes the new producer (ad valorem) tax.

According to statistics provided by China Tobacco,[4] the relative distribution of producer sales incomes in 2008 was about 20% for cigarettes with a producer price of 7 RMB per pack or more, 30% for those priced between 5 RMB and 7 RMB, and 50% for brands costing less than 5 RMB per pack. Since ad valorem tax revenue is based on the price of cigarettes, not the quantity sold by type, the value of sales is used to reflect the relative weights of government tax revenue received from different classes of cigarettes. Cigarette prices in China vary from about 2.0 RMB ($0.30) per pack to more than 200 RMB ($29.41) per pack.[5] Thus, the weighted ad valorem tax rate net increase in the producer price under the new adjustment is 11.7% $((21.9\% \times 0.2) + (-0.2\% \times 0.3) + (14.8\% \times 0.5))$.

Table 1:   Comparison of Chinese Tobacco Excise Tax Structure before and after 1 May 2009

	Before 1 May 2009	After 1 May 2009
Specific excise tax	0.06 RMB	0.06 RMB per pack
Ad valorem tax		
Price per pack	≥5 RMB 45%	≥7 RMB 56%
	<5 RMB 30%	<7 RMB 36%
Wholesale tax	0%	5%*

*Wholesale price includest he ad valorem tax.

The Chinese government has reported that the previous aggregate excise tax rate at the producer price level was 65%.[6] A 65% producer price tax rate translates to a retail price tax rate of 40%, $t_p/(t_p+1)$. With the new adjustment, our estimated 11.7% tax increase will increase the producer price tax rate to 76.7%. Thus, the new retail price tax rate will be 43.4% compared to 40%, an increase of 3.4%.

POTENTIAL IMPACT ON CHINESE GOVERNMENT TAX REVENUE, CIGARETTE CONSUMPTION AND POPULATION HEALTH

The new tax adjustment is focused on producer and wholesale prices. Since the Chinese cigarette industry is a national monopoly, the Chinese government has decided to absorb all of the tax increase. The government has predicted that this tax adjustment will generate an additional 50 billion RMB ($7.3 billion) in tax revenue.[7] We assume that this additional 50 billion RMB projected by the Chinese government is under the condition of no change in the retail price and, therefore, no change in cigarette consumption. Our new estimated adjusted rate at the producer price level (converting the new 5% wholesale price into producer price) is an additional 11.7% points. In 2008, the cigarette industry contributed4 50 billion RMB (in tax and profit) to the central government.[8] The 11.7% of 450 billion RMB is 52.65 billion RMB, which is quite close to the Chinese government forecast, showing that our estimated adjusted tax rate is quite consistent with the government projection.

Under the current Chinese government price policy, producers and wholesalers would not pass along these tax increases; thus, the tax increases will have no effect on cigarette consumption in China. While retail prices have not yet changed, consumers believe that the cigarette industry will eventually pass along these tax increases to the consumer.[9]

To simulate the potential impact of the recent tax adjustment if it were passed along to the retail level, we use 2007 baseline data since some of the key economic data for 2008 are not yet available. Below is a simulation assuming a 3.4% increase in the average price of cigarettes at the retail price level of 6.64 RMB ($0.98) per pack. Under the assumption of price elasticity of -0.15,[3] a conservative estimate, a 3.4% increase in the retail price will reduce cigarette consumption by about 545 million packs of the total national cigarette consumption of 106.98 billion packs. The government will gain an additional 22.58 billion RMB ($3.4 billion) in revenue. Based on the estimated participation (of quitting) elasticity of -0.06 (40% of -0.15 total price elasticity), with 308 million current smokers in China, an additional 3.4% tax increase will result in about 640 000 smokers quitting smoking and will avert 210 000 (one-third of 640 000) smoking related premature deaths among quitters.[10]

Under the assumption of price elasticity of -0.50, cigarette consumption would be reduced by 1.82 billion packs. Similarly, if the total price elasticity of the demand for cigarettes is -0.50, the participation (or quitting) price elasticity is -0.20. Under this simulation, an additional 3.4% tax increase in the retail price of cigarettes results in about 2.09 million of the 308 million current smokers in China quitting smoking, and 700 000 quitters (one-third of 2.09 million quitters) avoiding smoking-related premature deaths. The government will gain 19.63 billion RMB ($2.87 billion) in revenue.

The Chinese government's prediction of an additional 50 billion RMB in tax revenue from the new tobacco tax adjustment assumes no reduction in cigarette consumption. The recent shortfall of government tax revenue due to the economic down turn, coupled with the government's need to expand expenditures to stimulate the Chinese economy, requires additional tax revenue. The Chinese government has identified two sources of additional tobacco tax revenue: the announced increase in the ad valorem tax rate at the producer price level and the new additional 5% tax rate at the wholesale price level. These additional revenues will come from CNTC's profits as a monopoly. At present, because the tax burden has not been transferred to smokers, there is no price change for consumers, and thus, no public health benefit from the new tobacco tax adjustment.

CONCLUSIONS AND RECOMMENDATIONS

The motivation of the Chinese government with the recent tobacco tax adjustment is mainly to raise additional government revenue by adjusting its ad valorem tax on tobacco products. As shown from the revised tax structure, and allowing for no change in the retail price, the Chinese government intends to maintain its tobacco consumption sales and, in fact, its ad valorem tax will actually be reduced for the most mainstream price brands costing between 5 RMB and 7 RMB per pack. The government document makes no mention of whether this tobacco tax adjustment is related to China's compliance with the WHO Framework Convention in Tobacco Control (FCTC), Article VI. In response to comments from public health professionals concerning this recent Chinese government tobacco tax adjustment, the official China tobacco website indicates that the National Development and Reform Commission and CNTC are considering the possibility of transferring these tax burdens to consumers, particularly on the middle-lower price brands.[9]

The Chinese government could claim that this tax adjustment is a positive step towards the implementation of FCTC Article VI if these taxes are passed along to the retail price. The increase at the retail price level would be about 3.4%. Even with this relatively small tax adjustment, the projected impact would increase government revenue by between 19.63 billion to 22.58 billion RMB ($2.87 billion to $3.3 billion), reduce the number of smokers by between 640 000 and 2.09 million and reduce the number of premature deaths by between 210 000 and 700 000.

So far, this tax adjustment has left unchanged the relatively low specific excise tax on cigarettes (0.06 RMB per pack). The disadvantage of the ad valorem tax is that it creates incentives for smokers to switch to cheaper brands when taxes and prices rise, thereby reducing a potentially positive public health impact of a tax increase. In general, an increased specific excise tax is a most effective tax instrument for tobacco control, especially when the price of cigarette ranges so widely from about 2 RMB to more than 200 RMB per pack. Raising the specific excise tax would narrow the wide range of cigarette price dispersion in China. A specific excise tax is a cost-effective fiscal instrument that raises cigarette prices by the same amount across the board. The current two-tier ad valorem tax structure in China has, in fact, widened the gap between the two classes of cigarettes from 15% to 20% such that producers may be tempted to switch from higher prices to lower prices (setting the price below the Class A brand threshold to make it a Class B brand). Also the widening gap of the two-tier ad valorem tax may encourage smokers to switch to lower price brands, thus making the tax instrument less effective.

What this paper adds

- This paper provides an up-to-date policy analysis of the new Chinese tobacco tax rate adjustment.

We therefore recommend that the Chinese government raise the specific excise tax on cigarettes by additional 1 RMB per pack and eliminate the two-tier ad valorem tax, replacing it with a uniform tax rate. Since the Chinese government has just made a tax adjustment, it may not be realistic politically to change the tax structure in the immediate future. As a first step, therefore, we recommend that the Chinese government at least pass along the current tax increases from the producer/wholesale price to the retail price to fulfil its initial obligation to the FCTC. In the meantime, it is important for the tobacco control research community to evaluate the impact of the recent tax adjustment on potential changes in Chinese smoking prevalence, cigarette consumption patterns and industry responses.

ACKNOWLEDGEMENTS

The authors are grateful for the suggestions and comments provided by Dr Tom Frieden of the US Center for Disease Control and Prevention, Dr Frank Chaloupka of the University of Illinois, Chicago and anonymous referees of the journal. The authors remain responsible for the content of the paper, and the views expressed herein do not represent the authors' affiliations.

Funding US National Institutes of Health, Fogarty International Center Grant (R01-TW05938).

Competing Interest None.

Provenance and Peer Review Not commissioned; externally peer reviewed.

REFERENCES

1. China Ministry of Finance and State Administration of Taxation, May 26, 2009, http://www.shui5.cn/article/ct124017.html.
2. Shi J, Chen W . "Analysis of China's actual tobacco tax burden — a case study in Class A cigarette consumption tax." (In Chinese). In: Hu T, ed. *Tobacco taxation in China — history, current status, and reform.* Beijing: Chinese Finance and Economics Press, 2009.
3. Hu T, Mao Z, Shi J, *et al. Tobacco taxation and its potential impact in China.* Paris: International Union Against Tuberculosis and Lung Disease, 2008.
4. China National Tobacco Company, June 5, 2009, http://www.tobaccochina.com/news/analysis/wu/20074/2007416122_250334.shtml.
5. Zhang TQ. "Effects of tobacco consumption tax adjustment on brand competition." June 24, 2009. http://www.chinatobacco.com.

6. Liu T, Xiong B. *Tobacco economy and tobacco control* (In Chinese.). Beijing: Economic Science Press, 2004.

7. China National Tobacco Company, June 16, 2009. http://www.chinatobacco.com/20090812.

8. Beijing Review, 2009. http://www.bjreview.com.cn/business/txt/2009-07/04/content_205363.htm.

9. China National Tobacco Company, August 30, 2009. http://www.chinatobacco.com/20090830.

10. Shafey O, Ericksen M, Ross H, *et al. The tobacco atlas.* 3rd ed. Atlanta, GA: American Cancer Society, 2009.

Can Increases in the Cigarette Tax Rate be Linked to Cigarette Retail Prices? Solving Mysteries Related to the Cigarette Pricing Mechanism in China*

Song Gao, Rong Zheng and Teh-wei Hu

ABSTRACT

Objective To explain China's cigarette pricing mechanism and the role of the Chinese State Tobacco Monopoly Administration (STMA) on cigarette pricing and taxation.

Methods Published government tobacco tax documentation and statistics published by the Chinese STMA are used to analyse the interrelations among industry profits, taxes and retail price of cigarettes in China.

Results The 2009 excise tax increase on cigarettes in China has not translated into higher retail prices because the Chinese STMA used its policy authority to ensure that retail cigarette prices did not change. The government tax increase is being collected at both the producer and wholesale levels. As a result, the 2009 excise tax increase in China has resulted in higher tax revenue for the government and lower profits for the tobacco industry, with no increase in the retail price of cigarettes for consumers.

*Published in *Tobacco Control*, 2012; 21:560–562. doi: 10.1136/tobaccocontrol-2011-050027 (April 30, 2015).

Conclusions Numerous studies have found that taxation is one of the most effective policy instruments for tobacco control. However, these findings come from countries that have market economies where market forces determine prices and influence how cigarette taxes are passed to the consumers in retail prices. China's tobacco industry is not a market economy; therefore, non-market forces and the current Chinese tobacco monopoly system determine cigarette prices. The result is that tax increases do not necessarily get passed on to the retail price.

INTRODUCTION

On 9 January 2011, China entered its sixth year since signing the WHO Framework Convention on Tobacco Control (FCTC). To summarise and evaluate China's tobacco control progress in the past 5 years, an official assessment report titled *"Tobacco Control and China's Future"* was released recently.[1] The report's basic conclusion is that China has made limited progress towards tobacco control with poor performance in fulfilling its commitment to the FCTC. During the past 5 years, China has made some efforts with respect to non-price policies. These include instituting smoke-free public places and banning cigarette advertisement. However, China's tax and price measures have not been effective for tobacco control. The purpose of this paper is to discuss why the increased cigarette excise tax in 2009 did not lead to higher cigarette retail prices in China, uncover some of the mysteries behind the tobacco monopoly, describe the actual cigarette pricing mechanism and the role of the State Tobacco Monopoly Administration (STMA) on cigarette pricing and taxation.

In late May 2009, the Chinese Ministry of Finance and the State Administration of Taxation issued Taxation Legislation No. 84, *"The Notice Regarding Adjustment to Tobacco Product Excise Tax Policy"*,[2] effective 1 May 2009. The government stated that the purpose of the tax adjustment, which was an increase in the excise tax on cigarettes, was to increase government tax revenue from cigarettes and improve the tobacco tax structure in China, which was facing the pressure of both the worldwide financial crisis and tobacco control demands from WHO with respect to FCTC. It is interesting to note that tobacco control was not among the stated purposes of the tobacco tax adjustment.

Many people, especially tobacco control experts, expected that the increase in the excise tax rate on cigarettes would lead to increases in the retail price of cigarettes, given that tax and price increases have been widely proven the most effective measures for tobacco control worldwide in market economies.[3] But surprisingly and disappointingly, the STMA issued a document titled *Notice of Adjusting Cigarettes Allocation Price* (2009, No. 180),[4] also effective 1 May 2009, which declared that cigarette wholesale prices should remain the same nationwide as before the new excise tax adjustment. By maintaining wholesale prices, this regulation implied that the new tax policy would have no impact on cigarette retail prices. Because the Chinese tobacco industry does not operate under a market economy, the STMA could choose not to directly link the tax increase to cigarette retail prices in order to accomplish its political and social objectives. The connection between market forces and prices that lead to efficient allocation of resources in market economies does not operate in China.

The Chinese tobacco monopoly system affects cigarette prices in China, but exactly how it does so has remained a mystery. Unanswered questions include: Who determines cigarette prices in China? How many tiers are there within the cigarette pricing system? What is the actual cigarette pricing mechanism? The answers will help to explain why the 2009 tax adjustment did not change the retail price of cigarettes in China.

CHINA'S CIGARETTE PRICING MECHANISM — MYSTERIES AND ANSWERS

Mystery 1: Who Determines Cigarette Prices in China?

China's tobacco industry has adopted a system of unified leadership, vertical management and monopolised operation. The STMA and the Chinese National Tobacco Company are responsible for centralised management of staff, finance, properties, products, supply, distribution and domestic and foreign trade of the country's tobacco industry. The STMA manages the tobacco monopoly, and the Chinese National Tobacco Company, under the close supervision of the STMA, is responsible for marketing, production, distribution, sales and price setting of all cigarette products.

It is widely purported that either the National Development and Reform Commission (NDRC) or the tobacco industry itself decides cigarette prices in China. The NDRC is the ministry responsible for determining price policies of important commodities nationwide in China, and it supervised the tobacco industry from 2003 to 2008. Many people believe that the NDRC still has the power to influence cigarette prices. However, an examination of the tobacco monopoly law and related regulations in China reveals that the tobacco industry itself including cigarette factories, cigarette companies and tobacco monopoly authorities decide cigarette prices. The relevant major law and regulations include *the Law of the People's Republic of China on Tobacco Monopoly (1992 and 2009)*,[5] *Regulation of Macro-Adjustment and Administration on Cigarette Prices (STMA 1998, No. 108)*,[6] *Regulation on Cigarette Pricing (STMA 1998, No. 372)*[7] and *Notice of Strengthening Administration of Cigarette Prices (STMA 2000, No. 17)*.[8]

This tobacco monopoly law and regulations issued by the STMA explicitly state that the NDRC has no actual authority to decide cigarette prices, especially since 2008, when the Ministry of Industry and Information Technology took over the responsibility of supervising the tobacco industry from the NDRC. They also reveal that the STMA, which includes cigarette factories, cigarette companies and cigarette retailers, determines cigarette prices. Cigarette factories decide cigarette *producer price*; cigarette companies decide cigarette *wholesale price*; finally, cigarette retailers decide cigarette *retail price* by adding a regulated average market profit margin set by the STMA to the cigarette wholesale price. In other words, the STMA allows retailers to set their retail prices within a limited range, and these retail prices are monitored and reported to the STMA. All cigarette retailers operate under the licensure of the STMA.

Mystery 2: Is Producer Price the Tax Base for the Cigarette Excise Tax?

The tobacco industry in most countries has three tiers of cigarette prices: producer price, wholesale price and retail price. However, China's cigarette pricing system is composed of four categories: producer price, allocation price, wholesale price and retail price. Cigarette producer price consists of many complex components including raw material costs, labour costs, overhead costs, a variety of different taxes and another important component–profits. The costs and profits of cigarette manufacturers are confidential under China's tobacco monopoly, and it is impossible for outsiders, even the tax authority, to fully understand all the components. Producer price is not the tax base for the cigarette excise tax. Producer price is set by the cigarette factories. The tax base for cigarettes is the allocation price. The allocation price is the price negotiated between the STMA and the tax authority (i.e., State Administration of Taxation) and is based on producer price and kept as confidential industry information. The allocation price is officially used for tax collection purposes by the tax authority. In addition, the allocation price is used by the STMA for administration purposes as a classification criterion to categorise cigarettes from low-end to high-end for the purpose of tobacco monopoly administration.

Mystery 3: What is the Cigarette Pricing Mechanism?

The mystery of the cigarette pricing mechanism in China lies in the cigarette price formulation process. Under the current cigarette pricing process, the allocation price set by the STMA plays a pivotal role. It not only serves as a base for the tax rate and it also serves as a basis for setting wholesale price and retail price. The STMA also sets the profit margins for cigarette wholesalers (between allocation price and wholesale price, i.e., the allocation–wholesale profit margin) and for retailers (between wholesale price and retail price, i.e., the wholesale–retail profit margin). Given the allocation price, wholesale price is decided by adding the allocation–wholesale profit margin. Retail price is determined by adding the wholesale–retail profit margin to wholesale price. This pricing process implies that cigarette retail prices are under the control of the STMA because it can modify the cigarette allocation price and profit margins.

These profit margins figures are available to the public. Table 1 shows the allocation–wholesale profit margin and the wholesale–retail profit margin. The allocation–wholesale margin ranges between 15% and 34%. The wholesale–retail profit margin also is set by the STMA providing a limited range for retailers to follow (e.g., between 10% and 15%). Table 1 shows that there is a direct link among allocation price, wholesale price and retail price for different classes of cigarettes.

Mystery 4: Are the Profit Margins Declared by the STMA the Real Margins?

Even though data on all cigarette retail price/wholesale price and profit margins for different brand categories are available to the public, people still cannot figure out the cigarette allocation price correctly using such information. Thus,

Table 1:   Cigarette Profit Margins

Allocation Price Per Pack (RMB/Pack)	Between Allocation Price and Wholesale Price, %	Between Wholesale Price and Retail Price, %
[14.6, + ∞)	34	15
[10, 14.6)	29	15
[5, 10)	25	15
[3, 5)	25	10
[1.65, 3)	20	10
(0, 1.65)	15	10

Source: Notice of Adjusting Cigarettes Allocation Price (2009, No. 180) by State Tobacco Monopoly Administration.[4]
RMB, Renminbi (official currency of China).

the calculation of cigarette allocation prices is another mystery surrounding the tobacco industry in China. As a matter of fact, the officially announced allocation–wholesale profit margins (regulated profit margins) are not the actual margins. That discrepancy can explain why the tobacco monopoly keeps allocation prices an industry secret.

Using a set of unpublished government data provided by a provincial STMA bureau, we recalculated the margins and came up with the surprising finding shown below for the actual profit margins.

$$\text{Actual profit margin } (a') = \frac{\text{Regulated profit margin } (a)}{1 - \text{Regulated profit margin } (a)} \quad (1)$$

This equation shows that the actual allocation–wholesale profit margin increases along with the increased regulated profit margin. The recalculated margins are shown in Table 2. They show the true story about the profits from different classifications of cigarettes in China. We now understand why most cigarette producers are willing to produce high-priced (premium) cigarettes, which make much higher profits. These data reveal a different reality behind one of the mysteries of the Chinese tobacco industry.

Finally, the calculation of cigarette retail price can be demonstrated by the following formula:

$$\text{Pr} = A \times (1 + a') \times (1 + b) \times (1 + Rtvat), \quad (2)$$

Table 2: Cigarette Profit Margins (Regulated vs Actual)

Allocation Price Per Pack (RMB/Pack)	Regulated Allocation Wholesale Margin (a), %	Actual Allocation Wholesale Margin (a'), %
[14.6, + ∞)	34	51.52
[10, 14.6)	29	40.85
[5, 10)	25	33.33
[3, 5)	25	33.33
[1.65, 3)	20	25.00
(0, 1.65)	15	17.65

Source: Table 1 and estimated from equation (1).

where Pr indicates cigarette retail price, A represents allocation price (excise tax inclusive, *VAT* exclusive), a' is the actual allocation–wholesale profit margin, b is the wholesale–retail profit margin and *Rtvat* is the *VAT* rate. According to this equation, the allocation price, allocation–wholesale profit margin, wholesale–retail profit margin and *VAT* rate are the factors affecting the retail price of cigarettes.

Since the excise tax is collected at the producer level and wholesale level and not at the retail level, the effects of an increased excise tax on price can be absorbed by changing the allocation–wholesale profit margin $a(a')$. This is exactly what happened in 2009. The STMA significantly reduced the allocation–wholesale profit margin to coincide with the release of the new tobacco excise tax policy, and the wholesale price remained the same as before the tax adjustment. As a result, the 2009 excise tax increase in China has resulted in higher tax revenue for the government and lower profits for the tobacco industry, with no increase in the retail price of cigarettes for consumers. This relationship can explain why the 2009 excise tax policy adjustment did not change the retail price of cigarettes.

What this paper adds

This paper provides for the first time a detailed analysis of the Chinese tobacco pricing mechanism.

CONCLUSIONS

This paper has discussed the cigarette pricing mechanism in China and provided answers to some mysteries surrounding cigarette pricing in China's tobacco industry. We hope that the discussion will help the international tobacco control community understand the actual cigarette price formulation process in China and recognise that promulgating a tax rate increase is not sufficient to effect meaningful tobacco control in China. The 2009 tobacco tax adjustment in China provides an example of what happens when a tobacco monopoly company operating under government management pursues its political or social objectives that do not include an increase in the retail price. As can be seen in this paper, the Chinese tobacco monopoly can easily regulate allocation price and profit margins. The STMA does not subject to the market forces that influence prices in a market economy. If the Chinese tobacco industry can be separated from government ownership and established as a privatised enterprise, then taxation on cigarettes could be more effective in tobacco control since the likelihood of passing along the tax to the retail price could be increased. Alternatively, if the Chinese government decided to raise the retail price of cigarettes to consumers, either by instructing the STMA to directly raise prices or if the Ministry of Finance imposed a tax that the STMA passed through to retail price, then cigarette use in China would decrease.

ACKNOWLEDGEMENTS

We are grateful to Steve A. Tamplin for his support and encouragement of this study. We thank two anonymous reviewers for their very helpful comments and suggestions. All errors are our own.

Funding This study was supported in part by the Johns Hopkins Bloomberg School of Public Health, Bloomberg Initiative to Reduce Tobacco Use (SG and RZ), by the US National Institutes of Health, Fogarty International Center grant (R01-TW05938) and the Gates Foundation (T-wH).

Competing interests None.

Contributors Each author has contributed equally both in manuscript preparation and in data collection.

Provenance and peer review Not commissioned; externally peer reviewed.

Data sharing statement The authors would be glad to provide the data sources for Table 1 and Table 2.

REFERENCES

1. Yang GH, Hu AG. *"Tobacco Control and China's Future"*. Beijing: Economic Daily Publisher, 2011.
2. http://www.shui5.cn/article/cf/24017.html
3. World Bank. *Curbing the Epidemic: Government and the Economics of Tobacco Control.* Washington, DC: World Bank, 1999:23–35.
4. http://wendang.baidu.com/view/561db710cc7931b765ce1560.html
5. http://baike.baidu.com/view/88061.htm
6. http://www.tobacco.gov.cn/html/27/2701/270106/765274_n.html
7. http://www.tobacco.gov.cn/html/27/2701/270106/765278_n.html
8. http://www.tobacco.gov.cn/html/27/2701/270106/765289_n.html

The Potential Effects of Tobacco Control in China: Projections from the China SimSmoke Simulation Model*

David Levy, Ricardo L. Rodríguez-Buño
Teh-wei Hu and Andrew E. Moran

ABSTRACT

Objective To use a computer simulation model to project the potential impact in China of tobacco control measures on smoking, as recommended by the World Health Organization Framework Convention on Tobacco Control (FCTC), being fully implemented.

Design Modelling study.

Setting China.

Population Males and females aged 15–74 years.

Intervention Incremental impact of more complete implementation of WHO FCTC policies simulated using SimSmoke, a Markov computer simulation model of tobacco smoking prevalence, smoking attributable deaths, and the impact of tobacco control policies. Data on China's adult population, current and former smoking prevalence, initiation and cessation rates, and past policy levels were entered into SimSmoke in

---

*Published in *The BMJ*, 2014; 348. doi: 10.1136/bmj.g1134 (February 18, 2014).

order to predict past smoking rates and to project future status quo rates. The model was validated by comparing predicted smoking prevalence with smoking prevalence measured in tobacco surveys from 1996–2010.

Main outcome measures Projected future smoking prevalence and smoking attributable deaths from 2013–50.

Results Status quo tobacco policy simulations projected a decline in smoking prevalence from 51.3% in 2015 to 46.5% by 2050 in males and from 2.1% to 1.3% in females. Of the individual FCTC recommended tobacco control policies, increasing the tobacco excise tax to 75% of the retail price was projected to be the most effective, incrementally reducing current smoking compared with the status quo by 12.9% by 2050. Complete and simultaneous implementation of all FCTC policies was projected to incrementally reduce smoking by about 40% relative to the 2050 status quo levels and to prevent approximately 12.8 million smoking attributable deaths and 154 million life years lost by 2050.

Conclusions Complete implementation of WHO FCTC recommended policies would prevent more than 12.8 million smoking attributable deaths in China by 2050. Implementation of FCTC policies would alleviate a substantial portion of the tobacco related health burden that threatens to slow China's extraordinary gains in life expectancy and prosperity.

INTRODUCTION

China is the most populous nation in the world, and with over 50% of Chinese men smoking[1] accounts for about a third of the world's smokers.[2] China is also the world's largest tobacco producer, predominantly by government owned tobacco companies.[3] Reducing smoking in China would have an enormous public health impact, even on a global scale.

In 2003 China joined the World Health Organization Framework Convention on Tobacco Control (FCTC). The FCTC mandates a comprehensive set of tobacco control policies: surveillance and monitoring of the prevalence of tobacco use, creation of smoke-free environments, treatment of tobacco dependence, taxation on tobacco consumption and other price controls, and enforcement of health warnings on tobacco packages and marketing bans. China increased the tax on tobacco products at the producer and wholesale price level, with an average 11.7% increase in 2009. The tax increase did not, however, translate to higher retail prices experienced by consumers.[4] Of smoke-free environment regulations, only a smoking ban on public transportation has been legislated. China implemented treatment programs for tobacco dependence and to some extent bans on advertising, but these are weakly enforced. Overall, the country profile for China in the WHO 2011 report on the global tobacco epidemic identified multiple opportunities to improve implementation of the FCTC.[5]

Studies have estimated the health and economic burden of tobacco related diseases in China,[6–10] but none have estimated the potential health benefits of complete implementation of the FCTC. Using a version of the SimSmoke tobacco control policy model[11–18] populated with Chinese national demographic and tobacco exposure data, we projected the potential health impact of a comprehensive tobacco control program in China from 2015–50.

METHODS

The China SimSmoke Tobacco Policy Model

SimSmoke is a discrete-time first-order Markov process (state-transition) model of the prevalence of tobacco smoking and smoking related mortality that simulates the impact of tobacco control policies. The model begins in a baseline year, with the population divided into current, never, and former smokers by age and sex. The projected population is estimated using fertility and mortality data from the United Nations Population Division, Department of Economic and Social Affairs.[19] Smoking prevalence evolves with age and sex specific smoking initiation, cessation, and relapse rates. SimSmoke is programmed in Microsoft Excel (Office 2007 version; Microsoft, Redmond, WA, USA).

Tobacco Smoking Prevalence in China

We searched the WHO Global InfoBase for studies reporting sex and age specific prevalence of current smoking and ever smoking in China, inclusive of at least ages 15–74 years (see appendix and appendix Table 1).[20] The 1996 national prevalence survey provided estimates of current smoking prevalence for the simulation base year.[21] We estimated current smoking prevalence for specific ages by linear interpolation between midpoint ages for each 10 year age category.

In the 1996 survey, ever smokers were asked if they had quit. We estimated the prevalence of former smokers in 1996 as the difference between the prevalence of ever smokers and that of current smokers. Those who quit were further asked if they quit for less than six months, six months to one year, one to two years, and two years or more. We used these data to apportion the former smokers to groups representing less than one year, one to two years, and two years or more since quitting. Owing to lack of data for two years or more since quitting, we used US survey percentages (for 3–5 years, 6–10 years, 11–15 years, and ≥15 years) to apportion the former smokers who had quit for two years or more.[22]

Smoking rates evolve through age and sex specific initiation, cessation, and relapse rates. We assumed that cessation, initiation, and relapse rates depend only on current rates and not past behaviors (Markov assumption); that cessation and initiation rates are assumed constant over time, except when changes in policy occur; and that relapse rates are constant over time and unaffected by policies.

Owing to empirical challenges in measuring initiation and cessation among younger smokers and to ensure stability of the model, we measured initiation rates at each age as the difference between the smoking rate at that age year and the rate at the previous age year, determined by year at which smoking rates begin to level off. Because no similar data were provided in the global adult tobacco survey, we relied on the 1996 survey data for initiation and cessation rates. Based on an examination of prevalence data for 1996 and ensuing years, and 1996 data in the 1997 report showing stated ages of initiation,[2] prevalence rates increased until a specific age. Initiation in the model occurred until age 30 years for men and age 35 years for women. Cessation rates were based on published data in the 1997 report. Based on an examination of 1996 data on smokers who quit in the past year,[2] we set annual cessation rates in males equal to 2% for smokers aged 30–65 years and 3% for those ages 65 years or more. We set the cessation rates in females to 2%. We tracked cessation from age 30 years for males and age 35 years for females. Relapse rates were based on US rates, but the limited information provided on rates in China indicated that similar relapse rates applied. We adjusted first year relapse rates based on model calibration.

To calibrate and validate China SimSmoke predictions from 1996–2010, we used two surveys of tobacco use in China since 1996. The global adult tobacco survey, a cross sectional survey of tobacco use among adults in 16 low and middle income countries sponsored by the US Centers for Disease Control and Prevention and WHO, was used for age and sex specific current tobacco smoking prevalence in 2010 (see appendix).[23] We used six household survey waves from the multiprovincial China health and nutrition survey (repeated samples of the same households) to estimate the secular trend in active smoking prevalence from 1991 to 2006 (see appendix), with the first nine years used to calibrate the model.[24]

Relative Risk of All Cause Mortality in Current and Former Smokers

For all cause mortality we use relative risks of 1.35 for male smokers and 1.50 for female smokers aged 35–54 years, 1.35 for both sexes aged 55–64 years, and 1.30 for both sexes aged 65 years or more. Chinese studies that reported relative risks for all cause mortality in smokers compared with never smokers were in the range 1.19–1.40,[10,25–28] with most in the 1.30–1.40 range.[29] For former smokers, we assumed relative risks to decline over time at the rate observed in US studies.[30]

Tobacco Control Policies Simulated

We applied simulated policy effects to current smoking prevalence in the year in which the policy was or could be implemented, and, unless otherwise specified, applied to initiation and cessation rates in future years if the policy was sustained (Table 1). Unless synergies were specified, we reduced the effect of a second policy by [1 minus the effect of the first policy]. Except for the effects of cigarette prices and marketing bans, the model relies on studies of policy effects from high income countries, owing to the lack of studies for low and middle income countries. However, we considered two types of factors that may affect the impact of policies in low and middle income countries relative to high income countries; firstly, the degree of urbanization, which increases the potential reach and therefore effectiveness of policies. During the past 20 years, China's urban population increased from 18% to 46% of the total population.[31] A second factor is a population's baseline level of awareness of tobacco related harms. In countries with lower levels of income and general health awareness and no previous serious tobacco control campaigns, a lower base level of the knowledge of the dangers of smoking and of antismoking attitudes is expected to provide increased potential for the effectiveness of policies.

Table 1: Policies, Description, and Effect Sizes of SimSmoke Model and Policies in China

Policy	MPOWER Policy Simulated	Potential % Effect of MPOWER Policy	Current Policies in China
Tax policy	Cigarette price index adjusted for inflation for 1996 to 2010. Future prices increase with amount of cigarette tax in absolute terms of total taxes at 75% of retail price	Through price elasticity: -0.40 ages 15–17, -0.30 ages 18–24, -0.15 ages 25–34, -0.10 ages 35–64, and -0.15 ages ≥ 65	Tax rate of 40% was assumed at retail price. No tax change occurred from 2000–09. China specific price elasticities that vary by age are applied to the tracking period. Using these price elasticities, higher taxes are passed along to consumers, and applied to future active smoking prevalence
Smoke-free legislation:			
Worksite total ban	Ban in all areas	9.0% prevalence reduction effect	Smoke-free air laws are limited in China and determined at the municipal level, with no jurisdictions having a work ban (partial or limited) and relatively few private firms having their own bans (those few being international firms). No bans in restaurants, pubs, and bars; governmental facilities; educational facilities and universities; or healthcare facilities existed by 2010. Overall enforcement of regulation on smoke-free environments has been minimal
Restaurant and bar total ban	Ban in all indoor areas of restaurants	3.0% effect	
Other places total ban	Ban in 3 of 4 (malls, retail stores, public transportation, and elevators)	1.0% effect	
Enforcement and publicity	Government agency is designated to enforce and publicize laws. Publicity effect based on level of tobacco control funding	Effects weakened by as much as 50% if no enforcement and publicity	

Mass media campaigns:

Highly publicized campaign (well funded media and tobacco control campaign)	Meet requirements for medium level campaign, plus have per capita expenditures over $0.50 per capita from MPOWER, or evidence from other sources of strong, well focused media campaign and strong local campaigns	3.25% reduction (doubled when accompanied by other policies)	Low level media campaign, with no other policies in place
Low publicity campaign (low funded media and tobacco control campaign)	National agency and at least some level of funding and/or employees >0 from MPOWER, or evidence from other sources of intermittent media campaign	0.5% reduction (doubled when accompanied by other policies)	

(Continued)

Table 1: *(Continued)*

Policy	MPOWER Policy Simulated	Potential % Effect of MPOWER Policy	Current Policies in China
Marketing bans:			
Comprehensive ban	MPOWER: score 4. Ban on direct and indirect marketing. Ban applied to television, radio, print, billboard, instore displays, sponsorships, and free cessation samples	10.0% reduction in prevalence, 12.0% reduction in initiation, 6.0% increase in cessation	A "half way" policy between partial and complete advertising ban, with moderate enforcement (billboard and point of sale tobacco advertising is still allowed in China)
Weak ban	MPOWER: score 2. Partial ban on advertising. Ban applied to some of television, radio, print, and billboards	2.0% reduction in prevalence and initiation only	
Enforcement and publicity	Government agency designated to enforce laws	Effects weakened by as much as 50% if no enforcement	
Health warnings:			
Complete policy (strong health warnings)	MPOWER: score 4. Labels are large, bold, and graphic	1.0% reduction in prevalence, 1.0% reduction in initiation, and 5.0% increase in cessation rate	Weak health warnings enforced at same level over 1996 to 2010

Minimal policy (weak or minimal health warning)	MPOWER: score 2. Warning covers less than 30% of package, not bold or graphic	0.5% reduction in prevalence and initiation rates, 0.5% increase in cessation rate	
Cessation treatment policy	Complete availability and reimbursement of pharmaco and behavioral treatments, "quitlines," and brief interventions	6.75% reduction in prevalence, 55% increase in cessation	No information found on how long ago cessation treatments became available in China. Model assumed availability started in 2004
Access restrictions for youth strongly enforced and publicized	Compliance checks conducted regularly and publicized, penalties heavy, and bans on vending machines and self-service	30.0% reduction for age <16 years in prevalence and initiation only, 20.0% reduction for ages 16 and 17 in prevalence and initiation only	No minimum legal purchase age

MPOWER=simulated Monitor, Protect, Offer, Warn, Enforce, and Raise measures.
*Unless otherwise specified, same percentage effect is applied as percentage reduction in prevalence and initiation rate and percentage increase in cessation rate, and is applied to all ages and both sexes. Effect sizes are shown relative to absence of any policy.

The SimSmoke China base case (1996–2011) incorporated Chinese policies over the time period on tax policy, legislation on smoke-free environments, mass media anti-tobacco campaigns, bans on tobacco marketing, health warnings, cessation of treatment for tobacco dependence, and restrictions on access for youth. China SimSmoke simulated Monitor, Protect, Offer, Warn, Enforce, and Raise (MPOWER) measures,[32] a package of practical steps toward implementation of the FCTC, starting in 2012 and continuing through to 2050 (the last year projected by the model).

Model Outcomes

The two primary outcomes are annual smoking prevalence (percentage), and smoking attributable deaths by age and sex and all causes. From mortality rates, smoking prevalence, and relative risks we calculated the numbers of deaths by age, sex, and smoking status. We multiplied the number of current and former smokers at each age by their respective excess risk and summed the result to obtain total smoking attributable deaths. We compared the effect of implementing WHO FCTC/MPOWER measures in China starting in 2012, individually and in combination, with the status quo scenario in which tobacco control policies were maintained at 2010 levels. We then calculated the results for smoking prevalence in relative terms (percentage change in smoking prevalence compared with the status quo). The number of deaths averted was calculated as the difference between the number of smoking attributable deaths under the status quo and the number of smoking attributable deaths with policies implemented. Using 2005–10 China specific life expectancies estimated by the United Nations Population Division,[33] we tabulated life years lost at each age attributed to tobacco from life expectancies for the age at tobacco related death.

RESULTS

China SimSmoke Validation

Between 1996 and 2010, based on demographic projections, smoking initiation and cessation rates, and tobacco control policy effects, SimSmoke predicted that for ages 15 years or more, the prevalence of age standardized active smoking in males declined from 59.8% to 52.1% (see appendix Figure 1). The prevalence of active smoking in females declined from 3.5% to 2.4%. SimSmoke estimates of smoking prevalence in 2010 for ages 15 years or more were similar to the China global adult tobacco survey point estimate (52.9% for males; 2.7% for females) and within the survey's confidence interval boundaries (51.7% to 54.0% for males; 2.3% to 3.1% for females). In addition, SimSmoke projections fit well with active smoking trends in the China health and nutrition survey during 1991–2006. For younger ages (15–34 years), SimSmoke projections followed closely both the global adult tobacco survey 2010 estimate and the China health and nutrition survey trend. For older men and women (35–74 years), SimSmoke predictions mirrored the China health and nutrition survey trend but fell short of prevalence levels from the global adult tobacco survey. However, analyses of more specific age ranges (15–24, 25–44, 45–64, and ≥65 years) showed that all SimSmoke estimates for prevalence in 2010 fell within the 95% confidence intervals obtained by the China global adult tobacco survey, except for males aged 45–64 years (SimSmoke 59.1%; global adult tobacco survey range 60.0–65.8%, see appendix Table 2).

Projected Active Smoking Prevalence, China, 2015–50

Projecting the status quo scenario forward, active smoking in males was expected to decrease from 51.3% in 2015 to 46.5% by 2050 (Table 2⇩). The prevalence of active smoking in females was projected to decline slightly, from 2.1% in 2015 to 1.3% in 2050 (see appendix Table 3). In 2015, the estimated number of smoking attributable deaths alone was about one million (932,000 for males and 79,000 for females; totals, Table 3) and the estimated life years lost was about 14,562,000 (13,751,000 for males and 811,000 for females). In the status quo scenario, annual smoking attributable deaths in males were projected to increase through 2040 to about 1,459,000 but then decline to slightly less than 1.4 million by 2050. Projected annual life years lost reached about 17,029,000 by 2030 and then declined to 15,250,000 by 2050. Annual smoking attributable deaths in females were projected to be 49,000 in 2040 and 42,000 per year in 2050. Under current policies, a total of over 50 million smoking attributable deaths and 626,709,000 life years lost due to smoking were projected from 2012 to 2050 (Table 3).

Table 2:   Smoking Prevalence for Males Aged 15 to 85 Years in China, 1996–2050, Projected by the China SimSmoke Model (see Appendix Table 3 for Results in Females)

Projected Smoking Prevalence	1996	2010	2015	2020	2030	2040	2050
Smoking prevalence (%)							
Status quo policies	59.8	52.3	51.3	50.4	49.0	47.5	46.5
Independent policy effects:							
Tax at 75% of retail price	—	—	46.2	45.1	43.4	41.7	40.5
Comprehensive smoke-free air laws	—	—	46.7	45.7	44.3	42.7	41.7
Comprehensive marketing ban	—	—	49.7	48.7	47.2	45.6	44.6
High intensity tobacco control campaign	—	—	50.0	48.9	47.5	46.0	45.0
Strong health warnings	—	—	50.6	49.6	48.1	46.4	45.5
Youth access enforcement	—	—	51.0	49.9	48.3	46.6	45.5
Cessation treatment policies	—	—	49.9	48.8	47.1	45.5	44.6
Combined policy effects	—	—	35.4	33.6	31.4	29.4	28.2
% change in smoking prevalence from status quo							
Independent policy effects:							
Tax at 75% of retail price	—	—	−10.0	−10.5	−11.3	−12.2	−12.9
Comprehensive smoke-free air laws	—	—	−8.8	−9.2	−9.7	−10.1	−10.3
Comprehensive marketing ban	—	—	−3.0	−3.2	−3.6	−3.8	−4.1
High intensity tobacco control campaign	—	—	−2.6	−2.8	−3.0	−3.2	−3.3
Strong health warnings	—	—	−1.3	−1.5	−1.9	−2.2	−2.3
Youth access enforcement	—	—	−0.5	−0.9	−1.3	−1.8	−2.3
Cessation treatment policies	—	—	−2.7	−3.1	−3.8	−4.1	−4.0
Combined policy effects	—	—	−31.3	−33.8	−37.0	−39.6	−41.2

Status quo=scenario in which tobacco control policies were maintained at 2010 levels.

Impact of Implementing FCTC/MPOWER Measures

Relative to the status quo scenario, increasing cigarette taxes to 75% of the package price was projected to reduce smoking prevalence in relative terms by almost 10% for both sexes by 2015 (Table 2 and appendix Table 3). By 2050, smoking prevalence showed a relative reduction of 13% for males and of 12% for females in the taxation simulation. With a 75% tax, about 134,000 lives and 1,644,000 life years would be gained annually by the year 2050 (Table 3). Summing over the years 2015 to 2050, approximately 3.5 million deaths would be averted (3,333,000 for males and 143,000 for females) and 44,315,000 life

Table 3: Smoking Attributable Deaths and Life Years Lost in Males and Females Aged 15 to 85 Years in China, 2015–50, Projected by the China SimSmoke Model

Policy/Years	1996	2012	2015	2020	2030	2040	2050	2012–50
Status quo smoking attributable deaths	584,775	956,371	1,011,725	1,115,006	1,351,154	1,459,165	1,399,000	50,343,758
Premature deaths averted (change in smoking attributable deaths from status quo to policy implemented):								
Tax at 75% of retail price	—	—	20,525	43,945	110,905	123,413	133,815	3,476,341
Comprehensive smoke free air laws	—	—	17,698	40,032	110,954	126,329	127,803	3,437,409
Comprehensive marketing ban	—	—	11,314	25,307	69,539	78,523	80,421	2,149,873
High intensity tobacco control campaign	—	—	5,120	11,751	34,147	40,536	41,647	1,080,457
Strong health warnings	—	—	2,304	6,500	21,390	30,218	33,638	59,055
Youth access enforcement	—	—	—	—	63	1,150	2,977	27,186
Cessation treatment policies	—	—	5,221	15,346	51,416	73,327	79,800	1,825,782
Combined policy effects	—	—	62,059	142,725	400,924	475,113	494,191	12,765,972
Status quo life years lost	9,737,332	14,044,270	14,561,986	15,522,481	17,028,826	16,738,797	15,250,065	626,709,126

(*Continued*)

Table 3: *(Continued)*

Policy/Years	1996	2012	2015	2020	2030	2040	2050	2012–50
Life years gained (change in life years lost from status quo to policy implemented):								
Tax at 75% of retail price	—	—	281,268	597,457	1,424,838	1,547,173	1,643,770	44,315,184
Comprehensive smoke free air laws	—	—	263,877	579,045	1,415,029	1,470,649	1,422,007	42,103,017
Comprehensive marketing ban	—	—	168,961	368,444	900,977	948,680	948,726	27,138,822
High intensity tobacco control campaign	—	—	76,346	170,000	434,418	466,159	453,706	13,076,991
Strong health warnings	—	—	33,816	89,147	250,022	310,712	322,030	8,205,264
Youth access enforcement	—	—	0	0	2,559	43,226	92,598	949,533
Cessation treatment policies	—	—	76,130	206,643	580,247	705,141	686,079	18,582,968
Combined policy effects	—	—	903,791	2,015,417	5,040,733	5,490,093	5,479,588	154,247,987

Status quo=scenario in which tobacco control policies were maintained at 2010 levels.

years gained (42,882,000 for males and 1,433,000 for females) by the tax policy with the benefits continuing to grow in subsequent years.

Though increasing taxes had the largest impact on smoking prevalence, comprehensive smoke-free air laws and a well enforced marketing ban also showed potent and immediate effects. Comprehensive smoke-free air laws were projected to yield an almost 9% relative reduction in smoking rates by 2015, increasing to about a 10% reduction in 2050, and potentially averting about 3,437,000 deaths through 2050. A comprehensive marketing ban would reduce smoking prevalence by about 4.0% and avert 2.15 million deaths by 2050. A high intensity tobacco control campaign would lead to a 2.5% relative decline in smoking rates by 2015 and prevent about 1,080,000 smoking attributable deaths by 2050. Cessation treatment policies had smaller effects, with cessation policies growing over time to a 4% relative reduction. Stronger health warnings were projected to yield a relative 2.3% reduction in smoking rates by 2050.

When all MPOWER measures were combined, smoking prevalence was initially projected to decrease by about 30% relative to the status quo in 2015, and by about 40% by 2050. The model projected 494,000 (480,000 for males and 14,000 for females) fewer smoking attributable deaths by 2050 alone. By 2050, a total of approximately 12.8 million tobacco related deaths (12,274,000 for males and 491,000 for females) could be averted and 154,248,000 life years gained (149,303,000 for males and 4,945,000 for females) by implementing the complete set of policies.

DISCUSSION

Using the SimSmoke model calibrated to track with national estimates of smoking prevalence and repeated measures from a multiprovincial survey, we projected that complete implementation of the World Health Organization Framework Convention on Tobacco Control (FCTC)/Monitor, Protect, Offer, Warn, Enforce, and Raise (MPOWER) measures would lead to as much as a 34% relative reduction in male smoking prevalence by 2020, and a 41.0% reduction by 2050 (40 years after implementation). Despite the lag time expected between reductions in current smoking and declines in smoking attributable deaths, nearly half a million annual tobacco related deaths could be averted yearly by 2050. Without complete implementation of WHO

FCTC/MPOWER policies, and with other public health factors remaining unchanged, we projected that China will experience an additional 12.8 million preventable smoking related deaths and 154 million life years lost by 2050. Our projections suggest that the Chinese government's goal of less than 25% prevalence of active smoking in adults by 2015[34] is only achievable by adding to current tobacco control measures. The year 2025 goal of a relative 30% reduction in smoking prevalence in people aged 15 years and older targeted by WHO is achievable[35] but only with complete implementation of the WHO FCTC/MPOWER measures.

For many tobacco associated diseases (particularly chronic obstructive pulmonary disease and cancers) the risk related to tobacco use will not usually manifest until 20 years or more. Though we forecast decades into the future, given the "long shadow" cast by tobacco use, a 35 year simulation underestimates the impact of policies. Decreases in deaths related to second hand smoke from the direct impact of smoke-free air regulations and indirect impact of current smoking was not projected, leading to underestimation of the effects on smoking attributable deaths.

Taxation of tobacco products has been an effective means of tobacco control in many nations and was projected to be the most effective policy for China. Our results were broadly consistent with previous reports by one of the authors.[4,36,37] We assumed more sensitivity to price changes in younger smokers for several reasons. Teenage and young adult smokers generally earn lower wages, on average smoke less frequently (many less than daily), and are less dependent on tobacco than older smokers, all of which would lead to greater sensitivity to price increases. We also assumed fixed price elasticities over time. We considered an affordability index (price relative to income), but the model fit changes in trend better using a price (adjusted for inflation) index. However, in an economically rapidly developing nation where individual and household incomes have been rising rapidly, price increases may be increasingly more easily tolerated by smokers. In addition, we have assumed that tax increases will be passed along to consumers, leading to an increase in package price from 5.5 CNY ($0.90; £0.55; €0.66) to 13 CNY. A recent tax increase in China was absorbed at the producer (wholesale) level and resulted in no change on cigarette prices for consumers at the point of purchase.[4,38] However, if accompanied with other strong tobacco control policies, which reduce future demand for cigarettes and hence increase the incentive to increase current prices, large tax increases are more likely to lead to substantial if not commensurate increases in price. Our results show that multiple policy tools will be needed to substantially reduce the prevalence of smoking.

We projected that smoke-free air laws would be the second best policy, with all other policies simulated leading to more moderate projected effectiveness. As was the case years ago in other nations that evolved through the phases of the tobacco epidemic,[39] cigarette smoking is currently ingrained in Chinese cultural practices. The 2010 global adult tobacco survey found that many Chinese are largely unaware of the adverse health effects of smoking.[40] For this reason we modified our policy effectiveness assumptions for laws on a smoke-free environment, bans on marketing, and warnings on packaging to account for low awareness of the harms of tobacco in the adult population of China. In particular, the benefits of increasing awareness through health promotion are likely to play an increasingly important role in a country such as China where educational levels are increasing rapidly. Media campaigns can facilitate increased health awareness. The low rates for usage of cessation treatment and advice by health providers on the dangers of smoking also suggest an important role for the health sector, especially if cessation policies are combined with other policies.[41,42] Evidence indicates that many physicians in China smoke, and, given that physicians may be important role models, this practice should be strongly discouraged.[43,44] We allowed for synergies between media campaigns and other policies but may have underestimated policy effectiveness in assuming that the effect of adding a second policy is reduced if another policy is simultaneously implemented.

Strengths and Limitations of this Study

Though it is difficult to directly test the assumptions of China SimSmoke, we did incorporate nationally representative data on smoking prevalence and recent and historical tobacco taxation policies through price. Model validation showed that projections from 1996 to 2010 were consistent with the best available evidence on smoking prevalence levels (from the national surveys) and temporal trends (from the China health and nutrition survey). Inclusion of trend data from the China health and nutrition survey was particularly important for mitigating small variations in the different national surveys that may be due more to differences in survey design and sampling error than to temporal trends. In addition, SimSmoke has performed well in predicting smoking prevalence in over 20 countries, including comparison of model projections with historical effects of past implemented policies in other East Asian and middle income nations with widely different policies.[11–18,45–48] In particular, the Thailand and Korea models closely followed prevalence trends in nations with active tobacco control policies.[15,18] A SimSmoke analysis of tobacco control policies in Vietnam yielded results similar to those produced by a simulation modeling analysis of tobacco policies in Vietnam by Higashi and colleagues using a different approach.[48,49]

The model validated well, but our China projections should be interpreted with caution because to date evidence on policy intervention for the policies studied in the Chinese context is limited. Of all the policies, taxation has the best evidence base for low and middle income countries.[50] Evidence on the effectiveness of smoke-free laws on active smoking and media comes almost exclusively from high income countries.[51,52] In our analysis we incorporated China specific inputs wherever possible, including adjustments for a low population awareness of the harms of tobacco and the degree of urbanization. In other work, we have suggested that the percentage changes in smoking prevalence could vary by as much as 25% from our best estimate of the effect of changes in tax rates and by as much as 50% for the effects of other policies.[11,53]

Finally, data on cessation and initiation rates were generally not available over time and could not be validated over time. We conducted sensitivity analysis allowing cessation rates and initiation rates to vary by 10% from the levels used in the model. The resulting changes in smoking prevalence in males projected to 2050 were relatively robust, with ranges of 45.8% to 47.3% from variations in initiation rates and of 43.7% to 49.1% from variations in cessation rates. Given the low levels of cessation in 1996 and the low rates of advice to quit by healthcare providers and use of cessation treatment,[1] it will be important to monitor treatment use and cessation and initiation rates in the Chinese population.

Comparison with Other Studies

Our projections on status quo policy smoking attributable deaths for the years 2006 are similar to those estimated by Gu and colleagues.[10] Our projections for 2050 are, however, more conservative than Liu and colleague's prediction[27] of "about three million" smoking attributable deaths annually by that time, perhaps because they assumed no tobacco policy changes, and our status quo case incorporated effects of China's current tobacco control policies.

Conclusions and Policy Implications

Our estimates of China's burden of mortality attributable to smoking using the China SimSmoke tobacco policy model suggest that substantial health gains could be made — a 40% relative reduction in smoking prevalence and almost 13 million smoking attributable deaths averted and more than 154 million life years gained by 2050 — by extending effective public health and clinical interventions to reduce active smoking. Tax policies can play an especially important role, particularly if prices increase with taxes. Consistent with the WHO FCTC, smoke-free air policies, marketing restrictions, health warnings, media campaigns, and cessation treatment policies play an important role. Though smoke-free air laws and marketing bans require enforcement and some costs for implementation (including political capital), a recent report by WHO found that the policies suggested by the FCTC are clearly cost effective using traditional metrics,[54] a contention that has been reinforced by a study of tobacco control in Vietnam.[49] Studies of specific policies have also found that smoke-free air laws,[55] media campaigns,[56,57] and cessation treatment[58] are cost effective. Tax policy and health warnings, which involve minimal cost, are particularly cost effective.

In the next four decades, China will face over 50 million smoking attributable deaths, the largest absolute burden of smoking related deaths of any nation. Despite that the prevalence of smoking has been decreasing in China for both males and females, the absolute number of smokers will continue to increase for decades. This pattern of prevalence has been predicted globally: the 23.7% world's overall smoking prevalence for adults in 2010 will continuously decline to 22.7% by 2020 and to 22.0% by 2030, but the number of smokers will increase.[2] The consequences of inaction are considerable; without the implementation of the complete set of stronger policies, the death and disability legacy of current smoking will endure for decades in China.

ACKNOWLEDGEMENTS

We thank the government of the People's Republic of China for conducting the 1996 national prevalence survey and other national tobacco surveys, and the World Health Organization and US Centers for Disease Control for sponsorship of the global adult tobacco survey. This research uses data from the China health and nutrition survey. We thank the National Institute of Nutrition and Food Safety, China Center for Disease Control and Prevention; the Carolina Population Center, University of North Carolina at Chapel Hill; the National Institutes of Health (NIH; R01-HD30880, DK056350, and R01-HD38700); and the Fogarty International Center, NIH, for financial support for the China health and nutrition survey data collection and analysis files since 1989. We thank those parties, the China-Japan Friendship Hospital, and the China Ministry of Health for support for China health and nutrition survey 2009 and future surveys. Lastly, we thank the participants who contributed data to the surveys used for this research. DL received funding from the National Cancer Institute (NCI, 1R01TW009295-01) and Bloomberg Philanthropies to develop the China model and funding was received from the Cancer Intervention and Surveillance Modeling Network (CISNET) of the Division of Cancer Control and Population Sciences, NCI (grant UO1-CA97450-02) for general development of the SimSmoke model. T-WH was supported by the US Fogarty International Center of the National Institutes of Health and the National Cancer Institute of the National Institutes of Health (1R01TW009295-01). RLR-B was supported by a European Commission Erasmus Mundus masters program fellowship (Erasmus Mundus category A Europubhealth student scholarship, framework partnership agreement 2006-0047). AEM was supported by a US National Heart, Lung, and Blood Institute career development award (K08 HL089675-01A1).

Contributors: DL and AEM designed the study. DL designed and programmed the SimSmoke tobacco control model. DL and T-WH selected SimSmoke inputs for China. AEM and RLR-B designed the model calibration and validation method and reviewed and selected past Chinese tobacco surveys. AEM and RLR-B conducted original analyses of Global adult tobacco survey and China health and nutrition survey data. RLR-B ran all model simulations and prepared the results and produced the first draft of the manuscript. All authors contributed to writing and reviewing the manuscript. All authors had access to the SimSmoke model, original data, and approved of this manuscript. AEM and DL will act as guarantors.

Funding: This study was supported by Bloomberg Philanthropies; United States National Cancer Institute, National Heart, Lung, and Blood Institute, and Fogarty International Center; the European Commission. The funders took no part in the study design, study conduct, interpretation of the results, or preparation of the manuscript.

Competing interests: All authors have completed the Unified Competing Interest form at www.icmje.org/coi_disclosure.pdf (available on request from the corresponding author) and declare that RLR-B, AEM, T-WH, and DL have support from [the Bloomberg Philanthropies; United States National Cancer Institute, National Heart, Lung, and Blood Institute, and Fogarty International Center; and the European Commission] for the submitted work; have no relationships with any companies that might have an interest in the submitted work in the previous 3 years; their spouses, partners, or children have no financial relationships that may be relevant to the submitted work; and have no non-financial interests that may be relevant to the submitted work.

Ethical approval: Not required; all data analyses were secondary analyses of publicly available, de-identified data.

Data sharing: More details on the model data inputs and other assumptions are provided in a technical appendix. Researchers interested in using or exploring China SimSmoke software or development of a new national SimSmoke software version may contact the corresponding author at dl777@georgetown.edu.

Transparency: The senior author (DL) affirms that the manuscript is an honest, accurate, and transparent account of the study being reported; that no important aspects of the study have been omitted; and that any discrepancies from the study as planned have been explained.

What is already known on this topic

The prevalence of active smoking in Chinese men is among the highest in the world

Studies have estimated the mortality and disability burden attributable to smoking in China

They have not, however, estimated how much fully implementing measures recommended by the World Health Organization Framework Convention on Tobacco Control might change future smoking prevalence or prevent tobacco related deaths

What this study adds

Complete implementation of recommended tobacco control measures in China could lead to a relative reduction of over 40% in smoking and prevent almost 13 million tobacco related deaths by 2050

REFERENCES

1. Li Q, Hsia J, Yang G. Prevalence of smoking in China in 2010. *N Engl J Med* 2011;364:2469–70.
2. Mendez D, Alshanqeety O, Warner KE. The potential impact of smoking control policies on future global smoking trends. *Tob Control* 2013;22:46–51.
3. Yang GH, Ma JM, Liu N, Zhou LN. [Smoking and passive smoking, 2002]. [Chinese]. *Zhonqhua Liu Xing Bing Xue Za Zhi* 2005;26:77–83.
4. Hu TW, Mao Z, Shi J. Recent tobacco tax rate adjustment and its potential impact on tobacco control in China. *Tob Control* 2010;19:80–2.
5. World Health Organization. Report on the global tobacco epidemic, 2011: country profile China. www.who.int/tobacco/surveillance/policy/country_profile/chn.pdf.
6. Yang L, Sung HY, Mao Z, Hu TW, Rao K. Economic costs attributable to smoking in China: update and an 8-year comparison, 2000–2008. *Tob Control* 2011;20:266–72.
7. Lin HH, Murray M, Cohen T, Colijn C, Ezzati M. Effects of smoking and solid-fuel use on COPD, lung cancer, and tuberculosis in China: a time-based, multiple risk factor, modelling study. *Lancet* 2008;372:1473–83.
8. Zhang J, Ou JX, Bai CX. Tobacco smoking in China: prevalence, disease burden, challenges and future strategies. *Respirology* 2011;16:1165–72.
9. Wang JB, Jiang Y, Liang H, Li P, Xiao HJ, Ji J, *et al.* Attributable causes of cancer in China. *Ann Oncol* 2012;23:2983–9.
10. Gu D, Kelly TN, Wu X, Chen J, Samet JM, Huang JF, *et al.* Mortality attributable to smoking in China. *N Engl J Med* 2009;360:150–9.

11. Levy D, Zaloshjna E, Blackman K, Chaloupka F, Fong GT. The role of tobacco control policies in reducing smoking and deaths in the eighteen heavy burden nations: results from the MPOWER SimSmoke Tobacco Control Policy Model. In: Chaloupka FJ, Fong GT, Yurekli A, eds. The economics of tobacco and tobacco control. US National Cancer Institute Smoking and Tobacco Control Monograph 21. US Department of Health and Human Services, National Institutes of Health, 2014 (in press).

12. Currie LM, Blackman K, Clancy L, Levy DT. The effect of tobacco control policies on smoking prevalence and smoking-attributable deaths in Ireland using the Ireland SS simulation model. *Tob Control* 2013;22:e25–32.

13. Levy D, de Almeida LM, Szklo A. The Brazil SimSmoke policy simulation model: the effect of strong tobacco control policies on smoking prevalence and smoking-attributable deaths in a middle income nation. *PLoS Med* 2012;9:e1001336.

14. Levy DT, Boyle RG, Abrams DB. The role of public policies in reducing smoking: the Minnesota SimSmoke tobacco policy model. *Am J Prev Med* 2012;43(5 Suppl 3): S179–86.

15. Levy DT, Cho SI, Kim YM, Park S, Suh MK, Kam S. SimSmoke model evaluation of the effect of tobacco control policies in Korea: the unknown success story. *Am J Public Health* 2010;100:1267–73.

16. Levy DT, Nikolayev L, Mumford E. Recent trends in smoking and the role of public policies: results from the SimSmoke tobacco control policy simulation model. *Addiction* 2005;100:1526–36.

17. Nagelhout GE, Levy DT, Blackman K, Currie L, Clancy L, Willemsen MC. The effect of tobacco control policies on smoking prevalence and smoking-attributable deaths. Findings from the Netherlands SimSmoke tobacco control policy simulation model. *Addiction* 2012;107:407–16.

18. Levy DT, Benjakul S, Ross H, Ritthiphakdee B. The role of tobacco control policies in reducing smoking and deaths in a middle income nation: results from the Thailand SimSmoke simulation model. *Tob Control* 2008;17:53–9.

19. Saffer H. Tobacco advertising and promotion. In: Jha P Chaloupka F, eds. Tobacco control in developing countries. Oxford University Press; 2000:215–36.

20. World Health Organization. Non-communicable disease indicators database. 2012. http://apps.who.int/infobase/.

21. Yang G, Fan L, Tan J, Qi G, Zhang Y, Samet JM, et al. Smoking in China: findings of the 1996 national prevalence survey. *JAMA* 1999;282:1247–53.

22. US Bureau of the Census. Current population survey, 1992-93: tobacco use supplement file, documentation. 2012. http://riskfactor.cancer.gov/studies/tus-cps/info.html.

23. World Health Organization. Global adult tobacco survey. 2010. www.who.int/tobacco/surveillance/survey/gats/china/en/index.html.

24. University of North Carolina and Chinese Center for Disease Control and Prevention. China health and nutrition survey 1991–2006. 2012. www.cpc.unc.edu/projects/china.

25. Yuan JM, Ross RK, Wang XL, Gao YT, Henderson BE, Yu MC. Morbidity and mortality in relation to cigarette smoking in Shanghai, China: a prospective male cohort study. *JAMA* 1996;1646–50.

26. Chen ZM, Xu Z, Collins R, Li WX, Peto R. Early health effects of the emerging tobacco epidemic in China. A 16-year prospective study. *JAMA* 1997;278:1500–4.

27. Liu BQ, Peto R, Chen ZM, Boreham J, Wu YP, Li JY, *et al.* Emerging tobacco hazards in China: 1. Retrospective proportional mortality study of one million deaths. *BMJ* 1998;317:1411–22.

28. He Y, Chang Q, Huang JY, Jiang Y, Shi QL, Ni B, *et al.* [Study on mortality, incidence and risk factors of stroke in a cohort of elderly in Xi'an, China] [Chinese]. *Zhonghua Liu Xing Bing Xue Za Zhi* 2003;24:476–9.

29. Niu SR, Yang GH, Chen ZM, Wang JL, Wang GH, He XZ, *et al.* Emerging tobacco hazards in China: 2. Early mortality results from a prospective study. *BMJ* 1998;317:1423–4.

30. Shopland DR, Burns DM, Samet JM, eds. Changes in cigarette-related disease risks and their implication for prevention and control, smoking and tobacco control: National Cancer Institute, National Institutes of Health, 1997.

31. Henderson JV. Urbanization in China: policy issues and options. China Economic Research and Advisory Programme. Brown University and National Bureau of Economic Research, 2009.

32. World Health Organization. The MPOWER Strategy. 2012. www.who.int/tobacco/mpower/publications/en/index.html.

33. United Nations. Population Division Datasets. 2012. www.un.org/esa/population/unpop.htm.

34. General Administration of Quality Supervision, Inspection and Quarantine of the People's Republic of China. China Tobacco Control Programs 2012–2015. 2013. www.miit.gov.cn/n11293472/n11293832/n12843926/n13917012/15071046.html.

35. World Health Organization. Western Pacific Region Office (WHO-WPRO) global targets on Noncommunicable diseases. 2013. www.wpro.who.int/mediacentre/factsheets/fs20130311/en/.

36. Hu TW, Mao Z, Shi J, Chen W. Tobacco taxation and its potential impact in China. International Union Against Tuberculosis and Lung Disease, 2008.

37. Hu TW, Mao Z, Shi J, Chen W. The role of taxation in tobacco control and its potential economic impact in China. *Tob Control* 2010;19:58–64.

38. Li Q, Hu TW, Mao Z, O'Connor RJ, Fong GT, Wu C, *et al.* When a tax increase fails as a tobacco control policy: the ITC China project evaluation of the 2009 cigarette tax increase in China. *Tob Control* 2012;21:381.

39. Thun M, Peto R, Boreham J, Lopez AD. Stages of the cigarette epidemic on entering its second century. *Tob Control* 2012;21:96–101.

40. Center for Disease Control and Prevention. China global adult tobacco survey fact sheet. 12 Aug, 2010. www.who.int/tobacco/surveillance/en_tfi_china_gats_factsheet_2010.pdf.

41. Levy DT, Mabry PL, Graham AL, Orleans CT, Abrams DB. Reaching healthy people 2010 by 2013: a SimSmoke simulation. *Am J Prev Med* 2010;38(3 Suppl):S373–81.

42. Levy DT, Graham AL, Mabry PL, Abrams DB, Orleans CT. Modeling the impact of smoking-cessation treatment policies on quit rates. *Am J Prev Med* 2010;38(3 Suppl):S364–72.

43. Huang C, Guo C, Yu S, Feng Y, Song J, Eriksen M, Redmon P, Koplan J. Smoking behaviours and cessation services among male physicians in China: evidence from a structural equation model. *Tob Control* 2013;22(Suppl 2):ii27–33.

44. Jiang Y, Ong MK, Tong EK, Yang Y, Nan Y, Gan Q, *et al.* Chinese physicians and their smoking knowledge, attitudes, and practices. *Am J Prev Med* 2007;33:15–22.

45. Levy DT, Huang AT, Currie LM, Clancy L. The benefits from complying with the framework convention on tobacco control: a SimSmoke analysis of 15 European nations. *Health Policy Plan* 2013; published online 20 Nov.

46. Maslennikova GY, Oganov RG, Boytsov SA, Ross H, Huang AT, Near A, *et al.* Russia SimSmoke: the long-term effects of tobacco control policies on smoking prevalence and smoking-attributable deaths in Russia. *Tob Control* 2013; published online 12 Jul.

47. Ferrante D, Levy D, Peruga A, Compton C, Romano E. The role of public policies in reducing smoking prevalence and deaths: the Argentina Tobacco Policy Simulation Model. *Rev Panam Salud Publica* 2007;21:37–49.

48. Levy DT, Bales S, Lam NT, Nikolayev L. The role of public policies in reducing smoking and deaths caused by smoking in Vietnam: results from the Vietnam tobacco policy simulation model. *Soc Sci Med* 2006;62:1819–30.

49. Higashi H, Truong KD, Barendregt JJ, Nguyen PK, Vuong ML, Nguyen TT, *et al.* Cost effectiveness of tobacco control policies in Vietnam: the case of population-level interventions. *Appl Health Econ Health Policy* 2011;9:183–96.

50. Chaloupka FJ, Hu T, Warner KE, Jacobs R, Yurekli A. The taxation of tobacco products. In: Chaloupka FJ, Jha P, eds. Tobacco control in developing countries. Oxford University Press, 2000.

51. Callinan JE, Clarke A, Doherty K, Kelleher C. Legislative smoking bans for reducing secondhand smoke exposure, smoking prevalence and tobacco consumption. *Cochrane Database Syst Rev* 2010;4:CD005992.

52. Bala MM, Strzeszynski L, Topor-Madry R, Cahill K. Mass media interventions for smoking cessation in adults. *Cochrane Database Syst Rev* 2013;6:CD004704.

53. Levy DT, Hyland A, Higbee C, Remer L, Compton C. The role of public policies in reducing smoking prevalence in California: results from the California tobacco policy simulation model. *Health Policy* 2007;82:167–85.

54. World Health Organization. Scaling up action against noncommunicable diseases: how much will it cost? WHO, 2011.

55. Mudarri DH. The costs and benefits of smoking restrictions: an assessment of the SmokeFree Environment Act of 1993 (H.R. 3434). Environmental Protection Agency, Office of Radiation and Indoor Air, Indoor Air Division, 1994.

56. Hurley SF, Matthews JP. Cost-effectiveness of the Australian National Tobacco Campaign. *Tob Control* 2008;17:379–84.

57. Secker-Walker RH, Worden JK, Holland RR, Flynn BS, Detsky AS. A mass media programme to prevent smoking among adolescents: costs and cost effectiveness. *Tob Control* 1997;6:207–12.

58. Simpson SA, Nonnemaker JM. New York tobacco control program cessation assistance: costs, benefits, and effectiveness. *Int J Environ Res Public Health* 2013;10:1037–47.

The Consequences of Tobacco Tax on Household Health and Finances in Rich and Poor Smokers in China: An Extended Cost-Effectiveness Analysis*

Stéphane Verguet, Cindy L. Gauvreau, Sujata Mishra, Mary MacLennan, Shane M. Murphy, Elizabeth D. Brouwer, Rachel A. Nugent, Kun Zhao, Prabhat Jha, Dean T. Jamison

Summary

Background In China, there are more than 300 million male smokers. Tobacco taxation reduces smoking-related premature deaths and increases government revenues, but has been criticised for disproportionately affecting poorer people. We assess the distributional consequences (across different wealth quintiles) of a specific excise tax on cigarettes in China in terms of both financial and health outcomes.

Methods We use extended cost-effectiveness analysis methods to estimate, across income quintiles, the health benefits (years of life gained), the additional tax revenues raised, the net financial consequences for households, and the financial risk protection

*Published in March 13, 2015. doi.org/10.1016/S2214-109X(15)70095-1.

provided to households, that would be caused by a 50% increase in tobacco price through excise tax fully passed onto tobacco consumers. For our modelling analysis, we used plausible values for key parameters, including an average price elasticity of demand for tobacco of −0.38, which is assumed to vary from −0.64 in the poorest quintile to −0.12 in the richest, and we considered only the male population, which constitutes the overwhelming majority of smokers in China.

Findings Our modelling analysis showed that a 50% increase in tobacco price through excise tax would lead to 231 million years of life gained (95% uncertainty range 194–268 million) over 50 years (a third of which would be gained in the lowest income quintile), a gain of US$703 billion ($616–781 billion) of additional tax revenues from the excise tax (14% of which would come from the lowest income quintile, compared with 24% from the highest income quintile). The excise tax would increase overall household expenditures on tobacco by $376 billion ($232–505 billion), but decrease these expenditures by $21 billion (−$83 to $5 billion) in the lowest income quintile, and would reduce expenditures on tobacco-related disease by $24.0 billion ($17.3–26.3 billion, 28% of which would benefit the lowest income quintile). Finally, it would provide financial risk protection worth $1.8 billion ($1.2–2.3 billion), mainly concentrated (74%) in the lowest income quintile.

Interpretation Increased tobacco taxation can be a pro-poor policy instrument that brings substantial health and financial benefits to households in China.

Funding Bill & Melinda Gates Foundation and Dalla Lana School of Public Health.

INTRODUCTION

Many low-income and middle-income countries, such as China, have undergone an epidemiological transition from communicable to non-communicable diseases in recent years, which imposes a growing economic burden on these nations.[1,2] Tobacco use is a leading modifiable risk factor for non-communicable diseases, and in 2010 there were an estimated 5 million premature deaths attributable to smoking worldwide.[3] Asia has the highest number of tobacco users and is the prime target of tobacco companies.[4,5] Health behavioural changes have accelerated rapidly in China, including increasingly higher numbers of cigarettes smoked in the already very large male smoker population.[6] Furthermore, the prevalence of smoking in women is still relatively low.[7] In 2010, 1 million premature deaths were attributable to smoking in China, and the three leading causes of death (stroke, ischaemic heart disease, and chronic obstructive pulmonary disease) were linked to tobacco consumption.[8,9]

Tobacco taxation is widely recognised as very effective at reducing smoking, its attributable morbidity and mortality,[10] and subsequently the burden of non-communicable diseases.[3,11] Additionally, it provides revenues and potential for redistributive health financing.[4,12,13] Tax comprises about two-thirds of the retail price of cigarettes in most high-income countries but less than half of the total price in most low-income and middle-income countries such as China, which indicates that there is potential room for taxation as a fiscal and health policy instrument.[10,12,14−18]

Although tobacco taxation is a cornerstone of the WHO Framework Convention on Tobacco Control,[19] which was ratified by China in 2005, some controversy exists because of the potential regressivity of excise taxes such as those for tobacco. This regressivity is caused by the fact that poor people already spend a larger proportion of their income on smoking than do their wealthy counterparts, and taxes paid by the poor would constitute a larger proportion of their income than that of the rich,[20] which is a source of concern to policy makers.[21] Although a given tobacco tax could be viewed as progressive depending on the specific methods used to assess the tax burden and the data source used,[22] most researchers conclude that tobacco taxes exert a negative distributional effect. However, poor people are substantially more responsive to price changes than are their wealthy counterparts, which means that their consumption and tax burden could be lower,[21,23−25] and therefore policy might reduce regressivity.

The effect of tobacco taxation should also be considered alongside the fact that tobacco and tobacco-related disease expenditures exacerbate the effects of poverty. Excessive medical spending attributable to smoking and consumption spending on cigarettes combined were estimated to impoverish 55 million Chinese people in the late 1990s.[26] Smoking could also contribute to cycles of impoverishment if expenditures on education are displaced by those on smoking.[27−30]

In 2009, China launched a US$125 billion 3-year health reform plan, the goals of which included achievement of universal health coverage and prevention of medical impoverishment.[31] Since then, impressive progress has been made in provision of health insurance coverage, resulting in narrowing of the health care access gap between poorer and richer individuals. However, in one important area — financial risk protection — advances still need to be made because insurance covers only about 50% of inpatient costs and 30–40% of outpatient costs.[31,32] In 2011, the poorest quartile of households in China

Research in context

Evidence before this study

We did a search of PubMed using the search terms "China", "tobacco", "taxation", "impact", "socio-economic", "economic evaluation", "modeling", "income inequality", "youth", and "demand" in various combinations. We did not use any language or date restrictions. We did the same search on Google Scholar. We searched resources from relevant websites, especially from WHO and the International Agency for Research on Cancer. We also consulted with experts in the specialty.

Tobacco smoking is responsible for 5 million premature deaths worldwide. China has the highest number of tobacco users (>300 million) and is a prime target of tobacco companies. The deleterious health and economic consequences of smoking have been increasingly assessed and include modelling studies to identify suitable interventions. Tobacco taxation is widely recognised to be very effective at reducing tobacco use and initiation, and it provides financial revenues and potential for redistributive health financing. Tax comprises about two-thirds of the retail price of cigarettes in most high-income countries but less than half of the price in China, which indicates that there is potential room for taxation as a fiscal and health policy instrument. Few studies have assessed the distributional consequences of increased excise tobacco taxes in Asian economies, although the health and economic benefits of such a policy could be substantial.

Added value of this study

In this study, we used a unified analytical framework of extended cost-effectiveness analysis (ECEA) that models the distributional consequences (across income quintiles) in China of an increase in tobacco price of 50% through excise tax in terms of the health benefits (premature deaths averted), the additional tax revenues raised from excise tax, the net financial consequences for households, and the financial risk protection provided to households. We estimate substantial health gains, and find that reductions would occur in expenditures on tobacco-related disease, and financial risk protection from higher tobacco taxation; these benefits would disproportionally favour the lower-income population quintiles. We conclude that higher tobacco taxation can be a pro-poor policy device that brings substantial health and financial benefits to households in China.

Implications of all the available evidence

Higher tobacco taxes in China can reduce a substantial proportion of the global burden of smoking-related morbidity and mortality. Since tobacco use is a strong risk factor for many non-communicable diseases, for which health policy is still formulating in low-income and middle-income countries, large and immediate tax increases could have far-reaching health benefits, lower health care costs, and reduced disparities in health and economic outcomes, especially for the poorest populations. The estimation of financial risk protection of tobacco control policy is an especially fertile topic for further studies when considered in conjunction with the movement towards universal health-care coverage, which is gathering strong momentum in many countries.

had about twice as much catastrophic expenditure on health as those in the wealthiest quartile.[33]

Little work has studied the distributional consequences of increased tobacco taxation, although the health and economic benefits of such a policy could be substantial in Asian economies.[4] Previous studies have assessed the policy outcomes including health benefits, health-care costs, regressivity, and financial risk protection separately and with different analytical devices. Here, we use the analytical method of extended cost-effectiveness analysis (ECEA)[34] that can provide insights into these questions simultaneously in a unified model. We apply ECEA[34–36] to a hypothetical excise tax that would raise the retail price of cigarettes by 50% in China. In the Chinese male smoking population, we estimate the distributional consequences (across income quintiles) of this hypothetical excise tax in terms of: health benefits (years of life gained); additional tax revenues raised from the excise tax; net change in expenditures on both tobacco products and tobacco-related disease (e.g., stroke) treatment; and the financial risk protection provided to households by avoiding impoverishing health-care expenditures.

METHODS

Model

Our modelling approach draws substantially from the Asian Development Bank's framework[4] that estimates the effect of taxation-created cigarette price shocks. It accounts for price responsiveness across age and socioeconomic groups to compare the tax burden and health gains in each stratum based on existing and projected numbers of future smokers.[4] Since Chinese men comprise the vast majority (96%) of smokers in the country (53% of men are smokers vs 2% of women[37]), this study focuses solely on the male population, which we model for 50 years. The population is replenished as older individuals die. The population is divided into five age groups of smokers: those younger than 15 years of age (representing potential future smokers); 15–24-year-olds; 25–44-year-olds; 45–64-year-olds; and those older than 65 years. These groups are further divided into income quintiles. Specifically, these quintiles were defined from four income cutoff values dividing the population into five groups (Table 1).

We simulate a one-time excise tax fully passed onto consumers that results in the retail price of a pack of cigarettes increasing by 50%. We use a pre-increase tax rate (41% or US$0.30) and cigarette pack price (US$0.74) extracted from MPOWER 2011,[39] to capture an average tax and price per pack purchased. Many different cigarette brands with a wide price range are available in China.[15,56–58] Hence, any tax increase will only benefit poor people if designed to reduce the so-called switching down effect to cheaper cigarette brands.[3,4,10]

The introduction of the excise tax has five main consequences: it reduces the number of premature deaths and associated years of life lost because of tobacco through induced smoking cessation; it brings excise tax revenues as tobacco price increases and cigarette consumption changes; it affects the household expenditures on tobacco depending on the tobacco price increase and cigarette consumption changes; it decreases expenditures on the treatment of tobacco-related disease as a consequence of the reduction in tobacco-related disease burden; and it brings financial risk protection to households by preventing medical expenditures related to the treatment of tobacco-related disease.

First, we estimate the years of life gained as a consequence of the price increase, solely among those who quit. We assume no health benefits would arise from reduced consumption caused by price changes among continuing smokers. Upon quitting, smokers gain a particular number of years of life, depending on their age at cessation.[40] We express years of life gained as a function of age a at cessation. At present, China's mean male life expectancy is

Table 1: Inputs Used in the Modelling for the Tobacco Excise Tax Increase (50% Retail Price Increase) in China

	Value	Data Source
Size of male population in China	677 million	UN data;[38] authors' assumptions
Age group (years)		UN data[38]
<15	18%	
15–24	17%	
25–44	33%	
45–64	24%	
≥65	8%	
Smoking prevalence per age		Asian Development Bank[4] and
group (%)		WHO[37]
15–24	34%	
25–44	59%	
45–64	63%	
≥65	40%	
Relative smoking prevalence per		Authors' assumptions based on
income quintile		education levels in references[4,37]
Income quintiles 1–4	1.14-times average per age group	
Income quintile 5 (richest)	0.86-times average per age group	
Cigarette consumption (cigarettes		Authors' assumptions based on
per day) per income quintile		education levels in references[4,37]
Income quintile 1 (poorest)	15.6	
Income quintile 2	15.5	
Income quintile 3	13.8	
Income quintile 4	12.7	
Income quintile 5 (richest)	12.7	
Price per pack of 20 cigarettes (2011 US$)	$0.74 (before excise tax increase), $1.11 (after excise tax increase)	Asian Development Bank[4] and WHO[39]
Price elasticity of demand for cigarette per income group		See Table 3

(*Continued*)

Table 1:   (*Continued*)

	Value	Data Source
Distribution of tobacco-related disease mortality, by cause (%)		Global Burden of Disease Study 2010[9]
Chronic obstructive pulmonary disease	11%	
Stroke	46%	
Heart disease	23%	
Neoplasm	20%	
Years of life gained upon tobacco cessation, per age group		Authors' assumptions based on Asian Development Bank data,[4] Doll *et al.*,[40] and Jha *et al.*[41]
15–24 year-olds	10 years	
25–44 year-olds	9 years	
45–64 year-olds	6 years	
≥65 year-olds	3 years	
Tobacco-related disease treatment costs (2011 US$)		Based on several studies[42–50]
Chronic obstructive pulmonary disease	$2078	
Stroke	$2024	
Heart disease	$10 845	
Neoplasm	$13 626*	
Use of health care by tobacco-related disease (%)		Based on several studies[51–53] and authors' assumptions
Chronic obstructive pulmonary disease	33%	
Stroke	80%	
Heart disease	81%	
Neoplasm	50%	
Relative use of health care per income quintile		Authors' assumptions based on reference[54]
Income quintile 1 (poorest)	0.79-times average	
Income quintile 2	0.98-times averages	
Income quintile 3	1.00-times average	
Income quintile 4	1.08-times average	
Income quintile 5 (richest)	1.15-times average	

(*Continued*)

Table 1: (*Continued*)

	Value	Data Source
Fraction of health care costs reimbursed by insurance schemes (%)	50%	Authors' assumptions based on Yip *et al.*[31]
Individual annual income (2011 US$)		Income distribution based on gross national income per person of
Income quintile 1 (poorest)	<$1652	$4940 and Gini coefficient of
Income quintile 2	$1652–3075	0.42[42,55]
Income quintile 3	$3075–4850	
Income quintile 4	$4850–7645	
Income quintile 5 (richest)	>$7645	

*Note that although many neoplasms are affected by smoking (e.g., oesophageal, mouth, trachea, bronchial, and lung cancers), for simplicity, we associate here neoplasm treatment cost with lung cancer treatment cost because of the significance of lung cancers among neoplasms affected by smoking and data availability.

71 years,[59] and the number of years of life gained is assumed to be realised 71–*a* after cessation. The number of quitters at age a is related to the participation elasticity, which is assumed to be half of the total price elasticity of demand for tobacco. In other words, we assume that half of price increases affects smoking rates (participation elasticity), and the other half affects the consumption of non-quitters. This proportion is consistently represented in findings and assumptions from studies over 25 years.[10,25,60,61] The total price elasticity (hereafter referred to as the price elasticity) refers to the change in number of cigarettes purchased by a population when price changes, owing to both outright quitting and reduced consumption of cigarettes. The change in smoking-related premature mortality is the product of the change in price increase, the price elasticity, the net effect of half this price change on smoking prevalence, and the life-years gained in those who quit depending on their age at quitting. The future smoking prevalence of those currently younger than 15 years of age is assumed to be the current prevalence rate for those aged 15–24 years. The model assumes that no additional smoking initiation occurs in those aged 15 years and older. This approach is conservative because the prevalence for those 15–24 years old is likely to rise in view of the peak for those aged 25–44 years.[62] Additionally, we assume that the price elasticity is twice as large

in young populations (15–24-year-olds and future smokers [i.e., those <15 years old]) than in older smokers.[4,10,61] Young smokers are generally believed to be more price responsive than older smokers because compared with older smokers they have less disposable income, lower addiction levels, and are more responsive to peer pressure.[63,64] Recent reviews[10,61] assessing tobacco use in youths showed that they can be two to three times more responsive to price than older people, with estimated price elasticities between −0.50 and −1.20 (where −0.5 and −1.20 equal a 0.5% and 1.20% fall in demand for every 1% increase in price) in most high-income countries. Although little research has been done on youth smoking in low-income and middle-income countries, similar conclusions generally apply.[10] As a case in point, results from the Global Youth Tobacco Survey[65] suggest that the price elasticity might be −1.8[66] or even −2.2.[67]

Second, we estimate the additional tax revenues raised from the excise tax. The annual change is related to the change in cigarette consumption (which in turn is related to price elasticity), the change in excise taxes per pack (from US$0.30 to $0.67 here), and the number of smokers in a particular age group. Similarly, we estimate the net change in expenditures on tobacco, related to price elasticity, the change of price per pack (from $0.74 to $1.11), and the number of smokers in a given age group.

Third, we estimate the net change in expenditures on treatment of tobacco-related disease, following the reduced number of tobacco-related premature deaths. The number of premature deaths averted is estimated on the basis of the assumption that about 50% of smokers die of smoking-related illness and that this risk is reduced upon quitting by 97% in 15–24-year-olds, 85% in 25–44-year-olds, 75% in 45–64-year-olds, and 25% in those older than 65 years.[4,40,41] The Global Burden of Disease Study 2010 classifies deaths caused by tobacco smoking as a risk factor among 20 possible disease outcomes (appendix),[68] which are aggregated into the following four largest tobacco-related causes of death in China: stroke, ischaemic heart disease, chronic obstructive pulmonary disease, and neoplasms.[9] Subsequently, we attribute the share of the premature deaths averted from these four causes. Based on these causes, and accounting for the proportion of people who will seek formal health-care treatment (health-care use), we assign treatment-related costs, to which we deduce the share reimbursed by insurance. Although many neoplasms are affected by smoking (e.g., oesophageal, mouth, trachea, bronchus, and lung cancers), for simplicity, we associate neoplasm treatment cost with lung cancer treatment cost due to the significance of lung cancers in neoplasms affected by smoking and data availability.

Finally, we quantify the financial risk protection provided to the households related to the reduction in the risk of expenditures on the treatment of tobacco-related disease. We use a money-metric value of insurance as our financial risk protection metric, which has been described elsewhere[34] and is detailed in the appendix. The results are then aggregated by income quintile. Complete details of the model are given in the appendix. We used R statistical software (R 3.1.0) for all statistical analyses.

Model Parameters

Tables 1–3 present all model key inputs. When relevant and where available data allow, parameter values vary by income quintile. For example, smoking prevalence and intensity (cigarettes per day) increase marginally as income quintile decreases.[4,37] For simplicity and in view of the difficulty in extrapolating outcomes for the future in rapidly evolving China, we assume no price increases and no changes in household incomes and socioeconomic status over time after the one-time tobacco price increase.

One key driver of the analysis is the price elasticity by income quintile. Estimated Chinese price elasticities range from -0.01 to -0.84[15,58,69–76] owing to variations in datasets and estimation methods, and as reviewed by Hu and colleagues[15,58] can be classified into: high-end elasticities (around -0.80) as obtained from two time series and often cited for developing

Table 2: Assumed Number of Smokers (in Millions) by Age Group and Income Quintile, Before Excise Tax Increase

	Total	Income Quintile 1	Income Quintile 2	Income Quintile 3	Income Quintile 4	Income Quintile 5
≥65-year-olds	24	5	5	5	5	4
45–64-year-olds	97	20	20	20	20	17
25–44-year-olds	142	30	30	30	30	22
15–24-year-olds	43	9	9	9	9	7
Future smokers (i.e., <15-year-olds)	43	9	9	9	9	7

Table 3:   Assumed Price Elasticity of Demand for Cigarette by Age Group and Income Quintile

	Average	Income Quintile 1	Income Quintile 2	Income Quintile 3	Income Quintile 4	Income Quintile 5
≥65-year-olds	−0.38	−0.64	−0.51	−0.38	−0.25	−0.12
45–64-year-olds	−0.38	−0.64	−0.51	−0.38	−0.25	−0.12
25–44-year-olds	−0.38	−0.64	−0.51	−0.38	−0.25	−0.12
15–24-year-olds	−0.76	−1.28	−1.02	−0.76	−0.50	−0.24
Future smokers (i.e., <15-year-olds)	−0.76	−1.28	−1.02	−0.76	−0.50	−0.24

These values are the authors' assumptions based on several studies.[4,10,58,61] A price elasticity of −0.38 equals a 38% fall in demand for every 100% increase in price.

countries;[10,61] middle-range elasticities (between −0.50 and −0.60), as estimated in half of studies and often cited for middle-income and high-income countries;[10,61] and low-end elasticities (lower than −0.15), as estimated from recent studies.[15,58] The latter elasticities could be explained by the wide price variation (more than ten-fold) across cigarettes, which enables smokers to switch to cheaper cigarettes without quitting, and the rising affordability of cigarettes concomitant to the rapidly growing economy.[15,56,58] In our analysis, we use −0.38 as our price elasticity, which corresponds to the mean elasticity from all studies reviewed by Hu and colleagues.[15,58] In general, poorer populations, whether within a country or between countries, have higher price elasticities than do wealthier ones.[10] We assume that the poorest income quintile is the most price elastic; the other quintiles are progressively less price elastic (based on data from Hu and colleagues[58]).

Sensitivity Analysis

To increase the robustness of our findings, we first did a multivariate sensitivity analysis, in which we simultaneously varied several key parameters (e.g., price elasticity and treatment costs). For this purpose, we did Monte Carlo simulations ($n = 100,000$ trials) to capture uncertainty in treatment costs, health-care use, and price elasticity of demand for tobacco inputs. Uncertainty was included by sampling n values for each parameter to which we assigned a beta distribution (e.g., price elasticity and use) or a gamma distribution (e.g., cost; appendix p. 9). Finally, in the *n* samples, extraction of the 2.5 and 97.5 percentiles allowed 95% uncertainty ranges (URs) to be established.

Second, we did univariate sensitivity analyses. We varied the price elasticity and set it to −0.38 across all income quintiles. We also varied the increase in the retail price of a pack of cigarettes attributable to excise tax, and alternatively set it to 25% (price increase from $0.74 to $0.92) and 100% (from $0.74 to $1.48).

Role of the Funding Source

The funder of the study had no role in study design or data collection. SV and coauthors had full access to all the data in the study. SV and DTJ had final responsibility for the decision to submit for publication.

RESULTS

After 50 years of a 50% tobacco price increase in China, 231 million years of life would be gained (95% UR 194–268 million), of which 79 million (34%) would accrue to the lowest income quintile (Table 4). The additional tax revenues raised from excise tax would be US$703 billion (95% UR 616–781), $98 billion (14%) of which would be borne by the bottom income quintile, compared with $149 billion (24%) in the highest income quintile and 170 billion (21%) in the second highest income quintile (Table 4). Total expenditures on tobacco would increase by about $376 billion (95% UR 232–505); however, these expenditures would decrease by $21 billion (95% UR −83 to 52) in the bottom income quintile and would increase in the other four income quintiles, ranging from US$40 billion (95% UR −27 to 107) in the second income quintile to $135 billion (86–164) in the fifth income quintile (Table 4). The expenditures on treatment of tobacco-related disease would decrease by $24 billion (95% UR 17–26), $6.6 billion (27%) of which would be concentrated in the poorest quintile. The financial risk protection afforded would amount to about $1.8 billion overall (95% UR 1.2–2.3) and would also be concentrated ($1.3 billion [74%]) in the poorest quintile (Table 4). Short-term results (within 10 years) are also given in the appendix.

The annual health gains are increasing over time because the younger age groups (15–24-year-olds and future smokers) contribute more substantially to the years of life gained and face a higher price elasticity than do older smokers

Table 4:   Cumulative Results for the Tobacco Excise Tax Increase (50% Retail Price Increase) in China, After 50 Years

	Total	Income Quintile 1	Income Quintile 2	Income Quintile 3	Income Quintile 4	Income Quintile 5
Years of life gained (millions)	231 (194–268)	79 (61 to 96)	63 (45 to 80)	47 (30–65)	31 (16–51)	11 (2–27)
Additional tax revenues raised from excise tax						
2011 US$ billion	703 (616–781)	98 (60 to 142)	134 (93 to 175)	152 (114–187)	170 (134–200)	149 (119–167)
% of individual income	—	3.87%	2.10%	1.43%	1.03%	0.65%
Change in expenditures on tobacco						
2011 US$ billion	376 (232–505)	−21* (−83 to 52)	40 (−27 to 107)	89 (27–147)	132 (73–182)	135 (86–164)
% of individual income	—	−0.82%	0.63%	0.84%	0.80%	0.59%
Expenditures on tobacco-related disease treatment averted						
2011 US$ billion	24.0 (17.3–26.3)	6.6 (4.9 to 8.6)	6.9 (3.9 to 7.5)	5.3 (2.7–6.1)	3.7 (1.7–5.9)	1.5 (0.3–3.3)
% of individual income	—	0.26%	0.11%	0.05%	0.02%	<0.01%
Financial risk protection afforded[†] (2011 US$ billion)	1.8 (1.2–2.3)	1.3 (0.8–1.8)	0.3 (0.1 to 0.4)	0.1 (0.06–0.2)	0.1 (0.02–0.1)	<0.1 (0.00–0.03)

95% uncertainty ranges are indicated in parentheses. *A negative value implies expenditures on tobacco averted.

[†]Measured by a money-metric value of insurance.

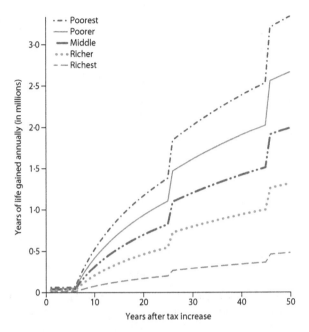

Fig 1: Annual Years of Life Gained for the Tobacco Excise Tax Increase (50% Retail Price Increase) in China, Over 50 Years, by Income Quintile

(Figure 1). The annual additional tax revenues from excise tax decrease over time as younger age groups, who are more price elastic than older people, replace older age groups and account for the majority of the population. The annual additional revenues raised start at US$17.7 billion per year (95% UR 15.5–19.7) in year 1, which accounts for about 15.9% of cigarette tax and industry profit and 1.2% of government revenue in China in 2011,[58,77,78] to eventually fall to $9.2 billion (8.0–10.3) in year 60, which represents about 8.3% of cigarette tax and industry profit and 0.6% of government revenue in China in 2011[58,77,78] (Figure 2). Finally, the annual change in expenditures on tobacco decrease over time as younger age groups, who are more price elastic than older people, replace older age groups and account for the majority of the population (Figure 3).

The paid out additional excise taxes represent a larger share of income of the low-income quintiles (3.9% and 2.1% for the bottom and second lowest income quintiles, respectively), than of the higher income quintiles (1.0% and 0.7% for the second highest and highest income quintiles, respectively;

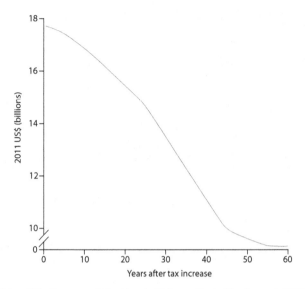

Fig 2: Additional Tax Revenues Raised by the Tobacco Excise Tax Increase (50% Retail Price Increase) in China, Annually, Over 60 Years

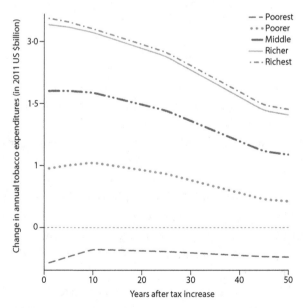

Fig 3: Annual Change in Expenditures on Tobacco, with the Tobacco Excise Tax Increase (50% Retail Price Increase) in China, Over 50 Years, by Income Quintile

A negative value suggests expenditures on tobacco averted.

Table 4). In terms of expenditures on tobacco, the lowest income quintile sees decreases in expenditures, representing −0.8% of their income, by contrast with the two highest income quintiles that see increases in expenditures on tobacco of 0.8% and 0.6% of their incomes, respectively (Table 4). Similarly, expenditures on tobacco-related disease averted as a fraction of income are higher in the bottom two quintiles (0.3% and 0.1%) than in the top two quintiles (0.02% at most). Therefore, in our base case scenario, although increased tobacco excise tax represents a larger share of income of the lower income quintiles, its other effects are largely positive and benefit poor populations disproportionately.

By contrast, when price elasticity is held constant at −0.38 across all income groups, the distributional consequences change substantially, as would be expected (Table 5). The health benefits are similar (47 million years of life gained) across all income quintiles apart from the fifth (35 million years of life gained), in view of the fact that smoking prevalence was assumed to be similar across the four quintiles, except for the fifth quintile (the richest quintile), which has a lower smoking prevalence than the other quintiles. Additionally, the bottom two income quintiles contribute to the additional tax revenues to a greater extent than the top two quintiles (Table 5). Furthermore, expenditures on tobacco increase for all income groups, with larger increases in the bottom two quintiles than the top two quintiles (Table 5). Finally, the expenditures on tobacco-related disease averted are evenly distributed across all income groups, between US$4 and $6 billion, although the financial risk protection afforded remains mainly concentrated in the poorest groups. In this latter scenario, tobacco taxation is more regressive, and the diminished benefits do not accrue as strongly to the lowest income groups, but nevertheless substantial financial risk protection is disproportionately achieved because of the decrease in tobacco-related health-care expenditures.

Finally, when retail price increase for a packet of cigarettes is set at $0.92 (25% price increase) or $1.48 (100% price increase), the distributional consequences for health benefits, expenditures on tobacco-related disease, and financial risk protection change only a little (although the overall changes are substantial). When cigarette packet retail price is $0.92, total health benefits are reduced to 115 million years of life gained, total expenditures on tobacco-related disease averted are reduced to $12.1 billion, and total financial risk protection provided to households falls to $0.9 billion. When retail price

Table 5:   Sensitivity Analysis Results (Cumulative) for the Tobacco Excise Tax Increase (Through Retail Price Increase) in China After 50 Years

	Total	Income Quintile 1	Income Quintile 2	Income Quintile 3	Income Quintile 4	Income Quintile 5
Price elasticity is set at −0.38 across all income quintiles						
Years of life gained (millions)	223	47	47	47	47	35
Additional tax revenues raised from excise tax						
2011 US$ billion	736	171	170	152	139	104
% of individual income	—	6.77%	2.67%	1.43%	0.84%	0.45%
Change in expenditures on tobacco						
2011 US$ billion	432	100	100	89	82	61
% of individual income	—	3.97%	1.56%	0.84%	0.49%	0.26%
Expenditures on tobacco-related disease treatment averted						
2011 US$ billion	24.9	4.1	5.2	5.3	5.7	4.6
% of individual income	—	0.16%	0.08%	0.05%	0.03%	0.02%
Financial risk protection afforded* (2011 US$ billion)	1.3	0.8	0.2	0.1	0.1	<0.1
Cigarette price is set at $0.92 (retail price increase is set at 25%)						
Years of life gained (millions)	115	39	31	23	16	6
Additional tax revenues raised from excise tax						
2011 US$ billion	421	74	87	89	93	78
% of individual income	—	2.93%	1.36%	0.84%	0.56%	0.34%

(Continued)

Table 5:   (*Continued*)

	Total	Income Quintile 1	Income Quintile 2	Income Quintile 3	Income Quintile 4	Income Quintile 5
Change in expenditures on tobacco						
2011 US$ billion	258	15	40	58	74	71
% of individual income	—	0.58%	0.63%	0.55%	0.45%	0.31%
Expenditures on tobacco-related disease treatment averted						
2011 US$ billion	12.1	3.3	3.5	2.7	1.9	0.7
% of individual income	—	0.13%	0.05%	0.03%	0.01%	<0.01%
Financial risk protection afforded* (2011 US$ billion)	0.9	0.7	0.1	0.1	<0.1	<0.1
Cigarette price is set at $1.48 (increase in retail price is set at 100%)						
Years of life gained (millions)	462	157	126	94	62	23
Additional tax revenues raised from excise tax						
2011 US$ billion	851	−5[†]	108	198	275	275
% of individual income	—	−0.21%[†]	1.70%	1.86%	1.66%	1.19%
Change in expenditures on tobacco						
2011 US$ billion	197	−242[†]	−80[†]	73	199	247
% of individual income	—	−9.6%[†]	−1.25%[†]	0.68%	1.20%	1.07%
Expenditures on tobacco-related disease treatment averted						

(*Continued*)

Table 5:   (*Continued*)

	Total	Income Quintile 1	Income Quintile 2	Income Quintile 3	Income Quintile 4	Income Quintile 5
2011 US$ billion	48.3	13.4	13.9	10.6	7.5	2.9
% of individual income	—	0.53%	0.22%	0.10%	0.05%	0.01%
Financial risk protection afforded* (2011 US$ billion)	3.6	2.6	0.6	0.2	0.1	<0.1

Three scenarios are assessed in this table: (1) price elasticity is set at −0.38 across all income quintiles (all other parameters remain identical as in the base case scenario); (2) increase in retail price of cigarettes is set at 25% (all other parameters remain identical as in the base case scenario, including price elasticity of demand for cigarette varying by income quintile); and (3) increase in retail price of cigarettes is set at 100% (all other parameters remain identical as in the base case scenario, including price elasticity of demand for cigarette varying by income quintile).

*Measured by a money-metric value of insurance.

†A negative value implies that expenditures on tobacco were averted.

is $1.48, total health benefits are increased to 462 million years of life gained, total expenditures on tobacco-related disease averted to $48.3 billion, and total financial risk protection provided to $3.6 billion. Nonetheless, we note variations for the additional revenues raised from excise tax and the net change in expenditures on tobacco. When the price of a cigarette pack is $0.92, the distribution of additional tax revenues raised remains almost unchanged: the bottom quintile contributes more substantially (in terms of income) than the other quintiles; however, it now sees an increase in tobacco expenditures. When the price of a packet of cigarettes is $1.48, the distribution of additional tax revenues raised changes substantially: the lowest income quintile sees a decrease in excise taxes paid and a substantial decrease in tobacco expenditures; the second lowest income quintile also undergoes a decrease in tobacco expenditures. In the 100% price increase, tobacco taxation is especially progressive: all health and financial outcomes provide substantial benefit to the poorest groups.

DISCUSSION

Tobacco tax hikes are essential in view of the increasing relative affordability of tobacco.[79,80] Since China's economy has grown enormously, cigarettes have become cheaper to smokers, which means that more aggressive tobacco taxation is now needed.

This study assesses the distributional consequences on four policy-relevant outcomes of a 50% retail price hike on tobacco products in China. Through the use of plausible values for key parameters, we find that in a 50-year period, in the male population, a 50% increase in tobacco price would lead to 231 million years of life gained (a third of these in the poorest group) and US$703 billion of additional tax revenues from excise tax (14% of this in the poorest group). It would increase overall household expenditures on tobacco by $376 billion, but reduce these expenditures by $21 billion in the poorest quintile; it would also decrease expenditures on tobacco-related disease by $24 billion (28% of which would be in the poorest group). Finally, it would provide financial risk protection worth US$1.8 billion, mainly concentrated (74%) in the poorest households. This situation means that tobacco taxation can be a pro-poor policy instrument that brings notable health and financial benefits to households and substantial revenues to society, which is especially important in the poor population of China, which has the highest number of smokers of any country worldwide.[3]

We also show that it is important to comprehensively integrate distributional aspects into analyses. We found that important insights into the equity of tobacco taxation can be otherwise missed when, as is done conventionally, a constant rather than an income-group-specific price elasticity is used. In China, where major reforms in health care are being made with the aim of reducing inequalities, proper assessment of policy instruments might be difficult unless explicit recognition of the income-specific variation in tobacco demand and health-care use and expenditures are made. In particular, Chinese price variation is more than ten-fold across different brands of cigarettes[15,56,58] as opposed to only about two-fold in most high-income countries,[3] which enables smokers to switch down with modest consumer tax increases.[80] Specifically, an effective price increase in China would need substantial increases in excise tax on the cheaper cigarettes[3,10] to narrow the large gap between cheap and more expensive cigarettes. The Indian Government, for example, has recently taken on cheaper cigarettes directly by raising the tax on lower end cigarettes more than that on more expensive brands. An important consideration is the weighing of taxation regressivity against the health benefits and financial risk protection resulting from reduced tobacco-related diseases in a consistent and similar framework such as here.

Our analysis has some limitations. First, uncertainty exists in the parameter inputs, of which the most important is the price elasticity of demand for tobacco. A wide range of elasticities has been estimated for China, and some studies have suggested that smokers in China could be quite insensitive to price changes compared with those in other countries.[81] We chose a middle value among the range of values for China, and one that is close to the accepted value for most countries (−0.4) and that would probably represent true price elasticities without the distortion of wide price variation that exists at present in China.[10] The wide variations in price including five classes of cigarettes[58] could change the brand selection of some smokers. Although we did not incorporate any such compensating behaviour (switching to lower price of cigarettes), as in Hu and colleagues' study,[15] we ran a sensitivity analysis with a low elasticity of −0.15, and noted that important health, additional excise tax revenues, and equity gains could still be realised (appendix p. 11). Although value-added taxes as in China's tiered price system encourage smokers to switch down to cheaper cigarettes, specific excise taxes as studied here can be designed to narrow the gap between cheap and expensive cigarettes to prevent smokers from swapping to cheaper brands.[15,58,80] Furthermore, we did a multivariate sensitivity analysis and our results were robust with the uncertainty imposed.

Second, we assumed that no health benefits would arise from reduced tobacco consumption because of a price hike among continuing smokers. Because we do not take into account the changes in the intensity of smoking, our estimates are therefore conservative. Similarly, we excluded female smokers from our analysis because they represent a small population (4% of all Chinese smokers[37]), although women's behaviour and household situation might somewhat differ from that of men.

Third, our epidemiological model has some shortcomings. For example, the non-linear harm caused by smoking intensity is not modelled.[82] Additionally, a more exhaustive dynamic model with, say, age-specific mortality with and without smoking would have yielded a more realistic and nuanced scenario, but simplicity of exposition, scarcity of data, and the benefits of transparency encouraged us to maintain our modelling approach. Furthermore, our results could have been discounted, treatment costs averted inflated using trends of the Chinese consumer price index, and individual incomes increased over the years with trends in the Chinese growth rate.[42] These adjustments would have unnecessarily complicated the results without providing any additional insight. Our financial analysis does not incorporate the effects of inflation and growth in gross domestic product and household income, which would ultimately strongly affect the benefits of tax increases of a fixed size. Neither does our model take into account consequences on tobacco consumers' utility, which is in any case ambiguous because of an (often) simultaneous willingness to pay for tobacco and for aid in cessation. Moreover, our model could have taken the household disposable income or used consumption data to estimate standards of living, but because of data shortcomings, gross national income distributed in income quintiles based on China's Gini coefficient was used as a substitute income indicator.[42,55] Likewise, we did not incorporate any perception of risks by individuals who smoke and the resulting effect on current consumption, or lagged consumption responses. Taxes could indeed serve as a self-control device to help reduce tobacco use and enable successful quitting.

Whether or not taxes are appropriately high depends in part on how excessively people underrate the harm from tobacco use.[83–86] However, these issues are not well explored in China or other low-income and middle-income countries, and extrapolation from studies done in high-income countries was judged to be inadvisable. Our analysis only focused on additional tax revenues raised from excise tax and did not estimate net government revenues through taxation. Since our intent is to take the consumer perspective, we did not model the Chinese tobacco tax structure. Indeed, China's tobacco industry operates under a system of monopoly that is able not to tie tax increases to cigarette retail prices.[16] Both a central government tax (e.g., value-added tax) and a local government tax (e.g., special tobacco leaf tax) are collected.[15,58] Hence, tobacco excise taxes will only have an effect when increases are passed onto the retail price.[16,80]

We show that it is possible and desirable to use the same framework to study distributional effects when a combination of outcomes related to different high-priority policy objectives need to be considered. This study shows that, despite potentially imposing a tax burden on low-income groups, tobacco taxation can bring substantial health benefits to poor people and can significantly reduce out-of-pocket expenditures for the poorest populations, especially as these lowest income groups are the most sensitive to increases in prices of tobacco products (panel). Increased tobacco taxation also brings significant financial risk protection to the poorest households through reductions in tobacco-related treatment expenditures.

More than 30 years ago the World Bank argued in support of Chinese government policies initiated in late 1981 to increase the retail price of cigarettes by 30%.[87] The current analysis has concluded that such policies are pro-poor in their financial as well as health consequences.

Contributors

SV and DTJ initiated and conceptualised the study. SV coordinated the research and did the analysis with CLG, SM, MM, SMM, and EDB. SV wrote the first draft of the report. RAN, KZ, PJ, and DTJ reviewed the report and provided advice and suggestions. SV and DTJ had final responsibility for the decision to submit for publication.

Declaration of interests

We declare no competing interests.

ACKNOWLEDGMENTS

We thank the Bill & Melinda Gates Foundation for funding through the Disease Control Priorities Network grant to the University of Washington. We received valuable comments from Evan Blecher, Zachary Olson, Clint Pecenka, Nisreen Salti, Helen Saxenian, and Gillian Tarr. Finally, we would like to thank five anonymous reviewers for providing very valuable and constructive suggestions.

REFERENCES

1. Bloom DE, Cafiero E, Jané-Llopis E, *et al.* The global economic burden of non-communicable diseases (no. 8712). Program on the Global Demography of Aging, 2012. http://ideas.repec.org/p/gdm/wpaper/8712.html (accessed April 20, 2014).
2. Jha P, Nugent R, Verguet S, Bloom D, Hum R. Chronic disease control and prevention. In: Lomborg B, ed. Global problems, smart solutions — costs and benefits. Cambridge: Cambridge University Press, 2013.

3. Jha P, Peto R. Global effects of smoking, of quitting, and of taxing tobacco. *N Engl J Med* 2014; 370: 60–68.

4. Asian Development Bank. Tobacco taxes: a win-win measure for fiscal space and health. Manila: Asian Development Bank, 2012.

5. Mackay J, Ritthiphakdee B, Reddy KS. Tobacco control in Asia. *Lancet* 2013; 381: 1581–87.

6. Yang G, Kong L, Zhao W, *et al.* Emergence of chronic non-communicable diseases in China. *Lancet* 2008; 372: 1697–705.

7. Ho MG, Ma S, Chai W, Xia W, Yang G, Novotny TE. Smoking among rural and urban young women in China. *Tob Control* 2010; 19: 13–18.

8. Yang G, Wang Y, Zeng Y, *et al.* Rapid health transition in China, 1990–2010: findings from the Global Burden of Disease Study 2010. *Lancet* 2013; 381: 1987–2015.

9. Global Burden of Disease Study 2010. Global Burden of Disease Study 2010. Results by risk factor 1990–2010. Seattle: Institute for Health Metrics and Evaluation, 2012.

10. International Agency for Research on Cancer, World Health Organization. IARC handbook of cancer prevention, volume 14: effectiveness of tax and price policies for tobacco control. Lyon: World Health Organization, 2011.

11. Jamison DT, Summers LH, Alleyne G, *et al.* Global health 2035: a world converging within a generation. *Lancet* 2013; 382: 1898–955.

12. Chaloupka FJ, Straif K, Leon ME. Effectiveness of tax and price policies in tobacco control. *Tob Control* 2011; 20: 235–38.

13. WHO. World Health Report 2010. Health systems financing: the path to universal coverage. Geneva: World Health Organization, 2010.

14. Jha P, Chaloupka FJ. Tobacco control in developing countries. New York: Oxford University Press, 2000.

15. Hu T-w, Mao Z, Shi J, Chen W. The role of taxation in tobacco control and its potential economic impact in China. *Tob Control* 2010; 19: 58–64.

16. Gao S, Zheng R, Hu T-w. Can increases in the cigarette tax rate be linked to cigarette retail prices? Solving mysteries related to the cigarette pricing mechanism in China. *Tob Control* 2012; 21: 560–62.

17. Hu T-w. Tobacco control policy analysis in China: economics and health. Singapore: World Scientific Publishing Co, 2008.

18. Levy D, Rodríguez-Buño RL, Hu T-w, Moran AE. The potential effects of tobacco control in China: projections from the China SimSmoke simulation model. *BMJ* 2014; 348: g1134.

19. World Health Organization. World Health Organization Framework Convention on Tobacco Control. http://www.who.int/fctc/en/ (accessed Dec 9, 2013).

20. Stiglitz J. Economics of the public sector, 3rd edn. New York: WW Norton & Co, 2000.

21. Warner KE. The economics of tobacco: myths and realities. *Tob Control* 2000; 9: 78–89.

22. Remler DK. Poor smokers, poor quitters, and cigarette tax regressivity. *Am J Public Health* 2004; 94: 225–29.

23. Chaloupka FJ. Rational addictive behavior and cigarette smoking, National Bureau of Economic Research Working Paper No. 3268. National Bureau of Economic Research, 1991. http://www.nber.org/ papers/w3268 (accessed April 20, 2014).

24. Townsend J, Roderick P, Cooper J. Cigarette smoking by socioeconomic group, sex, and age: effects of price, income, and health publicity. *BMJ* 1994; 309: 923–27.

25. Farrelly MC, Bray JW. Response to increases in cigarette prices by race/ethnicity, income, and age groups — United States, 1976–1993. *JAMA* 1998; 280: 1979–80.

26. Liu Y, Rao K, Hu T-w, Sun Q, Mao Z. Cigarette smoking and poverty in China. *Soc Sci Med* 2006; 63: 2784–90.

27. Wang H, Sindelar JL, Busch SH. The impact of tobacco expenditure on household consumption patterns in rural China. *Soc Sci Med* 2006; 62: 1414–26.

28. Xin Y, Qian J, Xu L, Tang S, Gao J, Critchley JA. The impact of smoking and quitting on household expenditure patterns and medical care costs in China. *Tob Control* 2009; 18: 150–55.

29. John RM, Ross H, Blecher E. Tobacco expenditures and its implications for household resource allocation in Cambodia. *Tob Control* 2012; 21: 341–46.

30. Hu T-w, Mao Z, Liu Y, de Beyer J, Ong M. Smoking, standard of living, and poverty in China. *Tob Control* 2005; 14: 247–50.

31. Yip W, Hsiao WC, Chen W, Hu S, Ma J, Maynard A. Early appraisal of China's huge and complex health care reforms. *Lancet* 2012; 379: 833–42.

32. Yip W, Hsiao WC. Non-evidence-based policy: how effective is China's new cooperative medical scheme in reducing medical impoverishment. *Soc Sci Med* 2009; 68: 201–09.

33. Meng Q, Xu L, Zhang Y, *et al.* Trends in access to health services and financial protection in China between 2003 and 2011: a cross-sectional study. *Lancet* 2012; 379: 805–14.

34. Verguet S, Laxminarayan R, Jamison DT. Universal public finance of tuberculosis treatment in India: an extended cost-effectiveness analysis. *Health Econ* 2015; 24: 318–32.

35. Verguet S, Murphy S, Anderson B, *et al.* Public finance of rotavirus vaccination in India and Ethiopia: an extended cost-effectiveness analysis. *Vaccine* 2013; 31: 4902–10.

36. Verguet S, Olson ZD, Babigumira JB, *et al.* Assessing pathways to universal health coverage in Ethiopia: health gains and financial risk protection afforded from selected interventions. *Lancet Global Health* (in press).

37. World Health Organization. Global Adult Tobacco Survey (GATS): China 2010 Country Report. Geneva: World Health Organization, 2010. http://www.who.int/tobacco/surveillance/gats/en/ (accessed Dec 9, 2013).

38. United Nations, Department of Economic and Social Affairs, Population Division. http://www.un.org/en/development/desa/population/publications/dataset/index.shtml (accessed Aug 13, 2013).

39. World Health Organization. MPOWER: a policy package to reverse the tobacco epidemic. Geneva: World Health Organization, 2011.

40. Doll R, Peto R, Boreham J, Sutherland I. Mortality in relation to smoking: 50 years' observations on male British doctors. *BMJ* 2004; 328: 1519.

41. Jha P, Chaloupka FJ, Moore J, *et al.* Tobacco addiction. In: Jamison DT, Breman JG, Measham AR, *et al.*, eds. Disease control priorities in developing countries, 2nd edn. New York: Oxford University Press and the World Bank, 2006.

42. World Bank. World development indicators. http://data.worldbank.org/data-catalog/world-development-indicators (accessed Dec 9, 2013).

43. She J, Yang P, Hong Q, Bai C. Lung cancer in China: challenges and interventions. *Chest* 2013; 143: 1117–126.

44. Le C, Zhankun S, Jun D, Keying Z. The economic burden of hypertension in rural south–west China. *Trop Med Int Health* 2012; 17: 1544–51.

45. Lee VW, Chan WK, Lam NL, Lee KK. Cost of acute myocardial infarction in Hong Kong. *Dis Manage Health Outcomes* 2005; 13: 281–85.

46. Wei JW, Heeley EL, Jan S, *et al*. Variations and determinants of hospital costs for acute stroke in China. *PLoS One* 2010; 5: e13041.

47. Ma Y, Liu Y, Fu H, *et al*. Evaluation of admission characteristics, hospital length of stay and costs for cerebral infarction in a medium-sized city in China. *Eur J Neurol* 2010; 17: 1270–76.

48. Heeley E, Anderson CS, Huang Y, *et al*. Role of health insurance in averting economic hardship in families after acute stroke in China. *Stroke* 2009; 40: 2149–56.

49. He QY, Zhou X, Xie CM, Liang ZA, Chen P, Wu CG. Impact of chronic obstructive pulmonary disease on quality of life and economic burden in Chinese urban areas. *Zhonghua Jie He He Hu Xi Za Zhi* 2009; 32: 253–57.

50. Zeng X, Karnon J, Wang S, Wu B, Wan X, Peng L. The cost of treating advanced non-small cell lung cancer: estimates from the Chinese experience. *PLoS One* 2012; 7: e48323.

51. Zhong N, Wang C, Yao W, *et al*. Prevalence of chronic obstructive pulmonary disease in China: a large, population-based survey. *Am J Respir Crit Care Med* 2007; 176: 753–60.

52. Zhao D, Liu J, Wang W, *et al*. Epidemiological transition of stroke in China twenty-one-year observational study from the Sino-MONICA-Beijing project. *Stroke* 2008; 39: 1668–74.

53. Chai Y, Xu H, Wang W, *et al*. A survey of factors associated with the utilization of community health centers for managing hypertensive patients in Chengdu, China. PLoS One 2011; 6: e21718.

54. Shanghai Municipal Center for Disease Control & Prevention (SCDC). Study on global AGEing and adult health (SAGE), Wave 1. China National Report. Study Report October, 2012. http://apps.who.int/healthinfo/systems/surveydata/index.php/catalog/13/download/ 1874 (accessed April 23, 2014).

55. Salem ABZ, Mount TD. A convenient descriptive model of income distribution: the gamma density. *Econometrica* 1974; 42: 1115–27.

56. Chinese Center for Disease Control and Prevention. Global adult tobacco survey (GATS) China 2010 country report. http://www.who.int/tobacco/surveillance/survey/gats/en_gats_china_report.pdf (accessed Dec 29, 2014).

57. Shang C, Chaloupka FJ, Zahra N, Fong GT. The distribution of cigarette prices under different tax structures: findings from the International Tobacco Control Policy Evaluation (ITC) project. Tob Control 2013; DOI:10.1136/tobaccocontrol-2013-050966.

58. Hu T-w, Mao Z, Shi J, Chen W. Tobacco taxation and its potential impact in China. Paris: International Union Against Tuberculosis and Lung Disease, 2008.

59. World Health Organization. Life tables. Global Health Observatory. http://www.who.int/gho/mortality_burden_disease/life_tables/life_tables/en/ (accessed Dec 9, 2013).

60. Gallet CA, List JA. Cigarette demand: a meta-analysis of elasticities. *Health Econ* 2003; 12: 821–35.

61. World Health Organization. WHO technical manual on tobacco tax administration. Geneva: World Health Organization, 2010.

62. Jha P, Jacob B, Gajalakshmi V, *et al*. A nationally representative case-control study of smoking and death in India. *N Engl J Med* 2008; 358: 1137–47.

63. Grossman M, Chaloupka FJ. Cigarette taxes, the straw to break the camel's back. *Public Health Reports* 1997; 112: 291–97.

64. Lewit EM, Coate D, Grossman M. The effects of government regulation on teenage smoking. *J Law Econ* 1981; 24: 545–49.

65. Global Youth Tobacco Survey Collaborative Group. Global Youth Tobacco Survey. http://www.who.int/tobacco/surveillance/gyts/en/ (accessed Dec 9, 2013).

66. Kostova D, Ross H, Blecher E, Markowitz S. Prices and cigarette demand: evidence from youth tobacco use in developing countries. National Bureau of Economic Research Working Paper No.15781. Cambridge, MA: National Bureau of Economic Research, 2010.

67. Nikaj S, Chaloupka FJ. The effect of prices on cigarette use among youths in the Global Youth Tobacco Survey. *Nicotine Tob Res* 2013; published online May 24. DOI: 10.1093/ntr/ntt019.

68. Lim SS, Vos T, Flaxman AD, *et al.* A comparative risk assessment of burden of disease and injury attributable to 67 risk factors and risk factor clusters in 21 regions, 1990–2010: a systematic analysis for the Global Burden of Disease Study 2010. *Lancet* 2012; 380: 2224–60.

69. Mao ZZ, Jiang JL. Demand for cigarette and pricing policy [in Chinese]. *Chinese Health Economics* 1997; 16: 50–52.

70. Hu T-W, Mao ZZ. Effects of cigarette tax on cigarette consumption and the Chinese economy. *Tob Control* 2002; 11: 105–08.

71. Mao ZZ, Hu T-W, Yang GH. New estimate of the demand for cigarettes in China. *Chin J Health Econ* 2005; 24: 45–47 [in Chinese].

72. Bai Y, Zhang Z. Aggregate cigarette demand and regional differences in China. *Appl Econ* 2005; 37: 2523–28.

73. Mao ZZ, Jiang JL. Determinants of the demand for cigarettes: a cross-sectional study. *Chin Health Service Management* 1997; 13: 227–29 [in Chinese].

74. Mao ZX, Yang GH, Ma H. Adults' demand for cigarettes and its determinants in China. *Soft Sci Health* 2003; 17: 19–23 [in Chinese].

75. Mao ZZ, Hu T-W, Yang GH. Price elasticities and impact of tobacco tax among various income groups [in Chinese]. *Chin J Evidence-Based Med* 2005; 5: 291–95.

76. Kostova D, Chaloupka FJ, Yurekli A, *et al.* A cross-country study of cigarette prices and affordability: evidence from the Global Adult Tobacco Survey. *Tob Control* 2014; 23: e3.

77. China Statistical Yearbook, 1989–2014. Beijing: China National Bureau of Statistics, 2014.

78. China Tobacco Statistics Yearbook, 1989–2014. Beijing: China National Tobacco Company, 2014.

79. Blecher EH, Van Walbeek CP. Cigarette affordability trends: an update and some methodological comments. *Tob Control* 2009; 18: 167–75.

80. White JS, Li J, Hu T-w, Fong GT, Jiang Y. The effect of cigarette prices on brand-switching in China: a longitudinal analysis of data from the ITC China Survey. *Tob Control* 2014; 23: i54–60.

81. Lance PM, Akin JS, Dow WH, Loh C-P. Is cigarette smoking in poorer nations highly sensitive to price? Evidence from Russia and China. *J Health Econ* 2004; 23: 173–89.

82. Schane RE, Ling PM, Glantz SA. Health effects of light and intermittent smoking: a review. *Circulation* 2010; 121: 1518–22.

83. Cherukupalli R. A behavioral economics perspective on tobacco taxation. *Am J Public Health* 2010; 100: 609–15.

84. Gruber J, Kőszegi B. Is addiction "rational"? Theory and evidence. *Q J Econ* 2001; 116: 1261–303.

85. Gruber J, Mullainathan S. Do cigarette taxes make smokers happier? *Top Econ Anal Pol* 2005; 5: 1538–653.

86. Gruber J, Kőszegi B. A modern economic view of tobacco taxation. Paris: International Union Against Tuberculosis and Lung Disease, 2008.

87. Jamison DT, Evans JR, King T, Porter I, Prescott N, Prost A. China, The Health Sector. Washington, DC: The World Bank, 1984.

Section IV

Tobacco Control in China: Barriers, Challenges and Recommendations

WHO Framework Convention on Tobacco Control in China: Barriers, Challenges and Recommendations*

Teh-wei Hu, Anita H. Lee and Zhengzhong Mao

ABSTRACT

Aim: The aim of this study was to analyze the barriers in the implementation of the Framework Convention on Tobacco Control (FCTC) in China and present recommendations on ways to address these challenges in tobacco control in China.

Methods: We review the available literature on progress and explore the barriers and challenges that impede a speedier pace in the adoption of the effective tobacco control measures, and present recommendations based on in-depth knowledge of decision-making process on the implementation of FCTC in China.

Results: The pace of progress in China is too slow. China faces intractable political, structural, economic and social barriers in tobacco control, which make the whole-hearted implementation of FCTC measures a painstaking process.

Discussion: The authors recommend a comprehensive approach to speed up the implementation of tobacco control measures. This includes strong political leadership from the top, structural changes to the tobacco industry and government oversight

*Published in *Global Health Promotion* 1757-9759, 2013; Vol 20(4): 13–22; 501910. doi: 10.1177/1757975913501910 http://ghp.sagepub.com.

of the tobacco industry, as well as advocacy and support for tobacco control from civil society at the grassroots level. (Global Health Promotion, 2014; 20(4): 13–22).

Keywords: tobacco, policy, advocacy, privatization

INTRODUCTION

The World Health Organization (WHO) Framework Convention on Tobacco Control (FCTC), with over 170 countries as signatories, is the first ever international treaty to address the tobacco epidemic and promote global public health. It provides a roadmap for effective tobacco control strategies to reduce demand for and restrict supply of tobacco products, and gives signatory countries a timetable to achieve specified milestones. Tobacco-related illness is a major component of the chronic diseases which cause a heavy human and economic toll. Tobacco control is thus a top priority in health promotion worldwide.

This is particularly true in China, where the smoking prevalence is high (1,2), the price of cigarettes is low and affordable (3), the mortality from smoking-related diseases is high (4), and the awareness level of the health risks of smoking is still relatively poor despite some improvements in the last 15 years (5). The country's 300 million smokers and 740 million men, women and children exposed to secondhand smoke are at risk of suffering from cancers, stroke, heart and respiratory diseases and other tobacco-related illnesses (6). The cost of smoking in China was estimated to have gone up 154% in direct costs and 376% in indirect costs in the eight years from 2000 to 2008 (7). This presents a significant challenge to China, a country which has made the epidemiological transition from infectious diseases to chronic diseases in a relatively short period of time as a result of the rapid economic development in the last few decades which brought about changing lifestyles (8).

Despite becoming one of the first signatories to the FCTC in 2003, the pace of tobacco control in China is very slow and results are lackluster at best. In WHO's ranking of the success of countries in tobacco control and FCTC compliance, China ranked in the bottom 20% (9). With so little to show since the country ratified the FCTC in 2005, there is a lot which needs to be addressed in order for tobacco control to really take root and become more effective as rapidly as possible.

This paper provides a framework for the analysis of the challenges and barriers in the implementation of the FCTC in China, as well as recommendations on how these challenges can be addressed. Views and suggestions presented here reflect the insights gleaned during the last decade by authors from discussions with senior political leaders in China's Ministries of Health, Finance, Agriculture, State Administration on Taxation, and a number of think tanks and policy research institutes.

THE TOBACCO ECONOMY

To understand the tobacco problem in China, an appreciation of the tobacco economy is essential. Tobacco is a state monopoly. China is by far the largest producer of tobacco in the world, producing 43% of the world total, which is more than the combined production of the next nine tobacco-producing countries (10). The China National Tobacco Company (CNTC) is the largest producer of cigarettes in the world, producing 2.375 trillion cigarettes in 2010 (11), a staggering 40% increase over the previous decade (12), and amounts to 41% of the world's total production in 2010 (10). Tobacco features significantly in government revenue, contributing in profits and taxes CNY 752.9 billion in 2011 (USD 118.5 billion, USD 1 = CNY 6.353 in Aug 2012) (13–15), amounting to 7.26% percent of government revenue (16). Furthermore, the livelihood of 20 million tobacco farmers (17), and millions more cigarette industry employees and over 300,000 cigarette retailers depend on tobacco farm subsidies, on growing tobacco leaf, on manufacturing jobs and on selling cigarettes for their livelihood (18). In tobacco leaf-growing provinces, more than half of the provincial government's revenue comes from tobacco. In the western province of Yunnan, for example, 77.8 percent of the provincial government's tax revenues in 2010 came from tobacco (19–21).

The importance of the tobacco economy in China cannot be overstated, and is therefore a very important political consideration among government leaders. Even though the harmful effects of smoking are now well known, and it has also been established that tobacco leaf farming causes environmental degradation, deforestation and harms the health of tobacco leaf farmers (22), government leaders view the continued growth of the tobacco industry as integral to the political and economic wellbeing of the country. As in many countries, achieving economic growth and political stability is the number one concern for political leaders in China, and tobacco control is not high on their list of priorities. The health consequences of smoking are considerations which are further out into the future than the tenure of most current political leaders. These considerations shape the attitude towards the country's tobacco control and FCTC implementation, and may explain the half-hearted efforts and minuscule resources that are devoted to it.

Of interest is the fact that the tobacco industry enjoys a certain amount of respectability in China, unlike its western counterparts. CNTC acknowledges that smoking is harmful and funds research to find 'healthier' alternatives for those who do smoke. Outreach activities, philanthropy and community building are also on their agenda, including activities for young people, building schools, and organizing health education seminars and academic conferences, etc. The general intention of CNTC's philanthropy is similar to that of any other tobacco company: to win public support and build a positive image (23). While such outreach and public interest activities are also conducted by many major international tobacco companies such as Philip Morris International and British American Tobacco, the CNTC has the advantage of being able to work directly with central and local governments, allowing the CNTC to provide funding for and to implement government collaborative projects such as building schools and improving local highways.

In the context of the size of the tobacco industry, these public interest and philanthropic projects constitute a minuscule percentage of the income of CNTC. Yet, all these programs help to justify the importance of the tobacco industry in the local community (24). A China Tobacco Museum in Shanghai is the largest such museum in the world. Built in 2004 and funded entirely by the industry, it is a shining example of the economic might and the social respectability the industry commands, and the length that it goes to in order to ensure the reach and continued prosperity of the industry.

BARRIERS TO EFFECTIVE TOBACCO CONTROL

Structural and Political Barriers

Examining where FCTC implementation is situated within the overall policy structure in the country is illuminating (Figure 1). Within the government structure, the highest powers reside with the National People's Congress. Power flows through the State Council to the relevant ministries: Health, Finance, Agriculture, Taxation, and Industry and Information Technology. The National People's Congress enacted the Tobacco Monopoly Law in 1991

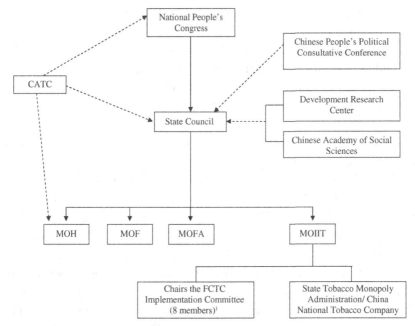

Fig 1: Organizational Chart for Tobacco Control Policy in China
Arrow: indicates the chain of decision-making.
Dotted Line: represents an advisory relationship.
MOF: Ministry of Finance.
MOFA: Ministry of Foreign Affairs.
MOH: Ministry of Health.
MOIIT: Ministry of Industry and Information Technology.
CATC: Chinese Association on Tobacco Control.
FCTC: Framework Convention on Tobacco Control.

[1]In addition to the four ministries shown, the other four members of the eight member committee are General Customs Administration, State Administration for Industry and Commerce, State Administration of Quality Supervision, Inspection and Quarantine, and the State Tobacco Monopoly Administration. The State Taxation Administration, Ministry of Agriculture, Ministry of Education, and Communist Youth League are no longer full members of the committee since 2011 but are brought into discussion as needed.

aimed at protecting the industry and establishing it as a monopoly (18). The State Council is advised by the Chinese People's Political Consultative Conference, the highest advisory mechanism in the country. The State Council gets policy inputs from its Development Research Center and the Chinese Academy of Social Sciences. CNTC falls under the jurisdiction of the State Tobacco Monopoly Administration (STMA), which is responsible for supervising the enforcement of the Tobacco Monopoly law and relevant laws and regulations. In practice, STMA the regulatory body and CNTC the industry are the same entity, with one management structure. STMA sets overall policies and delegates to CNTC full authority to implement these policies. STMA is under the Ministry of Industry and Information Technology (MOIIT) and has the goal of promoting the growth and stability of the tobacco economy (25–27). Thus both STMA and the industry itself have a strong stake to resist measures to implement FCTC.

The Chinese government has established an Inter-Agency FCTC Implementation Coordination Mechanism (ICM) in 2007 to implement the FCTC provisions. Currently, the ICM is made up of eight ministries which include the Ministry of Health (MOH), Ministry of Finance (MOF), Ministry of Foreign Affairs (MOFA) the MOIIT, as well as the STMA. Of interest is the fact that the ICM is established under the MOIIT, and not the MOH. The Minister of MOIIT holds the chairmanship. The tobacco industry is under the purview of the MOIIT, and therein lies an intrinsic problem: the MOIIT's role of spearheading the implementation of FCTC as chairman of the ICM is in direct conflict with its role as the ministry responsible for the management and development of the tobacco industry (28).

A good example of the ability of the state-owned industry to frustrate any tobacco control initiatives is the delay in implementing the warning labels on cigarette packages, as required by Article 11 of the FCTC. Years of wrangling took place among the MOH, the STMA, and the Chinese Association on Tobacco Control (CATC) which for a long time has been the only non-government organization devoted to tobacco control. The content and size of the new labels which resulted from such deliberations were found to comply with the letter, but not the intent, of the FCTC provision. Words of the health warning are in very small font size, or are in English, which is not understood by most smokers (29). Furthermore, graphic health warnings are considered inappropriate in the cultural context, as cigarettes are often given as gifts on auspicious occasions. Cigarette companies, both Chinese companies and transnational companies, are eager to exploit this with elaborate packaging of cigarettes to be used as gifts (30). As the STMA is a key member of the government's FCTC implementation committee, it can ensure that the measures taken cannot have the full effectiveness that is intended. New measures were introduced in April 2012 which called for larger font size and words to be in Chinese. The effectiveness of these new measures has yet to be studied. With regard to Article 15 of FCTC on restricted sales to minors, the legal minimum age to purchase cigarettes in China is 18. Enforcement of such a requirement among the hundreds of thousands of retailers is at best inconsistent.

With the tobacco economy enjoying such an important position, and with the industry well placed to protect its interests, tobacco control can be a politically sensitive topic. During the past 10 years, the authors have had numerous conversations at conferences as well as through personal contacts with senior officials from the administrative and legislative branches, research institutes and policy think tanks. Even though they are aware of the negative health consequences of smoking, these officials did not want to be unpopular among the vast smoking population. Nor are they keen to upset the status quo as far as the tobacco economy is concerned. Their unwillingness to champion the cause, or take an explicit policy stance on tobacco control, is a major barrier to the implementation of the FCTC.

ECONOMIC AND SOCIAL BARRIERS

Economically, the barriers to tobacco control are daunting. As mentioned earlier, the contribution of tobacco taxation to government revenue is significant, particularly so in tobacco leaf-growing provinces such as Yunnan, Hunan, Guizhou and Sichuan. Although research studies have demonstrated to the Chinese government, in particular MOF and State Administration for Taxation (SAT) officials, that raising tobacco tax would actually increase tobacco revenue despite a decrease in consumption, STMA is concerned that in the long run, the reduction of cigarette consumption would diminish the tobacco industry's contribution to the Chinese economy (3,31).

Contrary to the view held by senior policy leaders, empirical studies have shown that the potential negative impact of the reduction of cigarette sales on the employment of the tobacco industry and the livelihood of the tobacco farmers is not large, even for tobacco leaf-growing provinces. It has been shown that with an increase of CNY 1 (USD 0.1574) in the specific excise tax on a pack of cigarettes, which is estimated to lead to a 3.1 billion pack reduction in sales, the tobacco industry employment could lose about 1600 positions, assuming there is no opportunity for re-employment in the short run (3). Similarly, the income from tobacco farming is estimated to be reduced by CNY 260 million (USD 40.92 million), assuming there is no crop substitution (3). In reality, however, there are always opportunities in both the industry sector and the farming sector for alternative employment and crop substitution. Even though the positive health impact of reduced production will lead to one million lives saved (3), and any negative impact on employment and farming would only be minimal, the Chinese government has often used the negative aspect as an excuse not to raise tobacco tax. International studies have also shown that reduction in cigarette consumption would not reduce overall employment in the economy, as the switch from cigarette consumption to consumption of other goods and services would create additional employment (32).

Another concern in the minds of policy leaders is the inflationary pressure that an increase in cigarette prices may have. In reality, however, the weighting of cigarette prices in the basket of commodities measured in the consumer price index is very small, with alcohol and tobacco together contributing only 3.49% (19). Yet the perception of possible inflationary pressure presents a barrier to any effort to raise tobacco tax, one of the most effective tobacco control measures (33).

Perhaps one reason that economic considerations can feature so prominently in tobacco control considerations is the fact that smoking has long been an integral part of the country's social fabric. It is still a very acceptable social behavior, and serves as a social lubricant and connection builder. It enhances the daily social interactions of the smoker with his friends, boss and co-workers, as well as with relatives, all of whom very likely smoke (34). Offering cigarettes to friends is a symbol of friendship and a form of greeting, and gift giving of cigarettes is a common custom, particularly at festivals and celebratory occasions such as birthdays and weddings.

China's social norms apply not only to smokers, but also to non-smokers who seem to accept that it is inevitable that smokers will smoke in their presence. Awareness of health risks has been very low among non-smokers. As late as mid-2000, urban smokers in China considered that 'light' or 'low tar' cigarettes were less harmful than 'regular' or 'full flavored' cigarettes (35). The Global Adult Tobacco Survey in 2010 noted that only 23.2% of adults in China believe that smoking causes stroke, heart attack and lung cancer, and only 24.6% of adults in the country believe that exposure to tobacco smoke causes heart disease and lung cancer in adults and lung illnesses in children (2). Given that smoking and acceptance of smoking are social norms, and with these low levels of knowledge and awareness, social barriers to tobacco control in China are very challenging.

EQUITY ARGUMENTS IN TOBACCO CONTROL

Article 6 of the FCTC requires signatory countries to raise tobacco tax to discourage cigarette consumption. Political leaders in China subscribe to the commonly held belief that making cigarettes more expensive by raising tobacco tax places an unfair burden on low-income smokers and negatively impacts them disproportionately (32,36). It is no wonder that the government drags its feet in implementing this single most effective measure in tobacco control, despite the fact that this regressivity argument has to be seen in the context that such tax increase may be progressive from a public health standpoint. Larger reductions in smoking have been found to occur for those smokers in the lower income groups (37). The reluctance of the Chinese government to raise tax is evidenced by the fact that the 2009 tax adjustments involved a complicated reclassification of cigarette price levels and their corresponding tax rates, leading to a decrease in tax rates in cigarettes at certain price levels. Even such an adjustment led to considerable debate in the media about the fairness of it all (38).

Research in China has shown that expenditures on cigarettes constitute between 8 and 11% of total family expenditures in poor/near poor smoking households (39). Smoking households also spend less on food, housing, and education than nonsmoking households. Therefore, if households stopped buying cigarettes, these low-income smoking households could spend more money on essential goods. In addition to the negative impact of smoking on health, smoking also results in negative consequences in terms of human capital investment (40). The excessive medical spending attributable to smoking-related diseases and consumer spending on cigarettes has been estimated to be responsible for impoverishing 20 million residents in China during 1998 (41). Even though these evidence-based studies and research findings were published in major peer-reviewed journals, both English and Chinese, advocates still encounter challenges in communicating with top Chinese policymakers to disabuse them of the notion that raising tobacco tax is inequitable to the low-income population.

RECOMMENDATIONS TO CONFRONT THE CHALLENGES

China has unique characteristics when it comes to implementing the FCTC. These include the country's large population and number of smokers, national ownership of the tobacco industry, social and cultural backdrop and economic interest in the tobacco economy. During the past 10 years, numerous empirical studies have been published on the economic consequences of tobacco control in China, including the impact on government revenue, smoking prevalence, tobacco industry employment, and tobacco farming earnings. The evidence is there for a lot more to be done in tobacco control. Yet barriers persist. To overcome these barriers, the authors recommend a comprehensive strategy of top-down and bottom-up approaches. Figure 2 presents a conceptual framework in which policy leaders are influenced by a groundswell of popular support, and they in turn initiate changes that will benefit tobacco control.

Top-Down Approach

Under the current one-party political system, the central government has a clear mandate to set and implement overall national policy. The National People's Congress can enact legislative changes such as removing the Tobacco Monopoly Law. The Premier is the head of the Government, which is directly under the President who is the head of State and Chairman of the ruling party. It is a top-down administrative system which has proven to be very effective. Once the top officials have decided to implement a policy initiative, the country has a well-structured administrative apparatus. The handling of public health crises and natural disasters in recent years has shown that the administrative apparatus can work efficiently and effectively when there is a political will. A good example is the handling of the SARS (severe acute respiratory syndrome) epidemic in 2003 (42). Therefore, the critical success factor to tobacco control in China is top-level government leadership.

It is the authors' view that the change in the top leadership in China which has just taken place in March 2013 provides a golden opportunity for new impetus in tobacco control. This once-in-a-decade change of leadership has ushered in a new generation of leaders in China. They are younger and have grown up in an era of reform and opening in China, and are more open to Western ideas and values. History has shown that each new leadership has

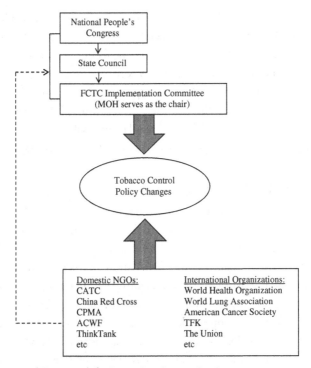

Fig 2: Conceptual Framework for Removing Current Barriers
CATC: Chinese Association on Tobacco Control.
CPMA: Chinese Preventive Medicine Association.
ACWF: All-China Women's Federation.
ThinkTank: ThinkTank Research Center for Health Development.
TFK: Campaign for Tobacco Free Kids.
The Union: International Union against Tuberculosis and Lung Disease.

sought to make their mark by initiating a new philosophy and new initiatives that seek to improve the wellbeing of the people. Tobacco control advocates should seize this window of opportunity to fight for an increase in tobacco tax, the most effective part of the tobacco control toolkit. Of importance is the need to link any tax increase to the retail price of cigarettes. Another important tobacco control measure that the new leaders can use to demonstrate that they really have the intent to control the tobacco epidemic is to initiate legislation to enforce the smoke-free regulations, with hefty penalties for those who do not comply.

It is therefore very important to provide these new top leaders with scientific evidence on policy impacts, costs of smoking, and benefits of tobacco control. In recent years, tobacco control advocacy from public health experts, civil society and international organizations, as well as current international trends, has resulted in top Chinese leaders feeling the need to take the moral high ground of supporting tobacco control more openly. Reaching and convincing this cohort of new leaders, especially those in MOF and SAT, to use price control measures such as tobacco taxation, and non-price control measures such as smoke-free rules and regulations, will go a long way towards overcoming the many barriers to tobacco control in the country.

Bottom-Up Approach

As shown in Figure 2, impetus for change can come from below as well. Even though China has 300 million smokers, non-smokers still outnumber smokers. Experience in many countries has shown that the tipping point in the battle against tobacco comes when non-smokers become aware that passive smoking is harmful to their health and that they have a right to a smoke-free environment. A groundswell of popular sentiment can be effective in influencing top leaders. Civil society, with non-governmental organizations, opinion leaders and other advocates can be a catalyst for change. Other countries have shown that civil society can play a significant role in advocacy, coalition building, providing evidence-based information, and being a watchdog as well as providing services such as smoking cessation counseling (43). There is currently only a handful of non-government organizations (NGOs) working on tobacco control in China, notably the CATC. With funding from international organizations, the CATC has been able to become more proactive in organizing educational and intervention programs in tobacco control, cultivating opinion leaders, and communicating with members of the National People's Congress, the highest legislative body, and the Chinese People's Political Consultative Conference, the highest advisory body. Furthermore, other NGOs such as the Chinese Red Cross and the All-China Women's Federation as well as academic bodies such as the Chinese Preventive Medicine Association have begun to devote efforts in recent years to tobacco control as part of their mission. The formation and involvement of more grassroots organizations to advocate for non-smokers' rights will be a step in the right direction. At the same time, international organizations such as the WHO, the World Lung Association, American Cancer Society, Red Cross, the International Union against Tuberculosis and

Lung Disease and philanthropic organizations such as the Gates Foundation and Bloomberg Initiative are supporting projects and building competencies in China.

With the increasingly prevalent use of internet technology among the population, these organizations take advantage of the social media and web technology as well as the mainstream media to increase knowledge of the health risks of active and passive smoking, and to raise the awareness of non-smokers to their right to smoke-free air in public places. The momentum for change from the community level will provide policy leaders at the top with many incentives to take action and to make more effective use of the tools in the tobacco control toolkit.

Structural Change

The major economic conflict for the Chinese government concerning implementation of the FCTC provisions is the government ownership of the tobacco industry and the STMA and CNTC being one and the same entity. With market-oriented activities and modern concepts of government oversight and monitoring increasingly becoming features of the Chinese economy, separating the tobacco industry from its regulatory state agency would be a step in the right direction. This will also move towards the goal of privatization of the tobacco industry. Two potential factors could lead the Chinese government to privatize the tobacco industry. First, with the growth of the Chinese economy, the role of the tobacco industry in terms of its economic contribution to central government revenue has been declining, as evidenced by the decreasing share of the industry's profit and tax contribution to central government revenue. Second, since China joined the World Trade Organization, transnational tobacco companies have become increasingly active in the Chinese cigarette market. Chinese tobacco economics research committees have begun to study whether the Chinese cigarette industry will become a 'sunset' industry in the future. Top government officials also have been looking at examples of the privatization of the cigarette industry in foreign countries, such as in Korea, Thailand and Turkey. The MOH and the CATC have begun officially endorsing the idea of withdrawal of government ownership and the transfer of CNTC to the private sector. Having the CNTC as a private entity would most likely result in a reduced direct economic conflict of interest for the government, and make it less able to resist the implementation of FCTC provisions. Such a fundamental structural change will need to be achieved through the National People's Congress, which can legislate the necessary changes to the Tobacco Monopoly Law. At the level of the ICM, changing the leadership of the committee from the MOIIT to the MOH will elevate the emphasis placed on health as the most important consideration in the implementation of the FCTC.

The structural change of privatizing the tobacco industry will also have ramifications for tobacco farming and address tobacco control from the supply side. Currently CNTC controls the sources of leaf production, allocation of leaf quotas and cigarette marketing channels. The CNTC has been subsidizing tobacco farmers and imposing a tobacco leaf tax as a source for local government revenue to ensure that the government can enforce the quota for CNTC (44). With a structural change, a private market for tobacco will enable farmers to switch to other crops which may be more lucrative. Pilot experiments of crop substitution for tobacco farmers to grow other cash crops has shown that this leads to increased output per acre and increased income for the farmers (17).

CONCLUSION

It is clear that China faces many barriers and major challenges to the effective implementation of tobacco control measures under the FCTC. In the past 7 years since the ratification of the FCTC, the Chinese government has yet to show its determination to give full effort to implement tobacco control measures in the country. Achievements are few and results dismal. With China becoming an increasingly visible player on the world stage, and being looked upon as having the resources to address problems to promote the health and wellbeing of its own people, it is incumbent upon the new leadership to show that there is the political will to tackle this problem. Separation of the STMA and the CNTC into distinct entities as regulator and industry respectively will be a first step towards privatizing the tobacco industry. Raising tobacco taxation and linking such tax increase to the retail price of cigarettes will reduce consumption, improve health and save lives. A national law to enforce smoke-free public place regulations with hefty cash penalties will go a long way towards protecting non-smokers from exposure to secondhand smoke.

China has the dubious distinction of having the largest number of active and passive smokers in the world, the largest area of farmland for tobacco leaf production and is the world's largest cigarette manufacturer. Success in addressing the tobacco problem in China would significantly decrease the global burden of tobacco-related illnesses and death, and promote global health. A comprehensive formula of strong political leadership, growing grassroots movements, increasing community awareness and changing social norms, coupled with structural changes to the tobacco industry to dislodge it from the entrenched position of power are essential ingredients to meet the challenges of tobacco control in China.

Conflict of Interest None declared.

Funding This research was supported by the Fogarty International Center and the National Cancer Institute of the United States National Institutes of Health under Award Number RO1 TW009295 and RO1 TW005938. The content is solely the responsibility of the authors and does not necessarily represent the official view of the National Institutes of Health.

REFERENCES

1. Li Q, Hsia J, Yang G. Prevalence of smoking in China in 2010. *N Engl J Med.* 2011; 364(25): 2469–2470.
2. World Health Organization. Global Adult Tobacco Survey (GATS) Fact Sheet China. 2010.
3. Hu TW, Mao Z, Shi J, Chen W. The role of taxation in tobacco control and its potential economic impact in China. *Tob Control.* 2010; 19(1): 58–64.
4. Gu D, Kelly TN, Wu X, *et al.* Mortality attributable to smoking in China. *N Engl J Med.* 2009; 360(2): 150–159.
5. Yang Y, Wang JJ, Wang CX, Li Q, Yang GH. Awareness of tobacco-related health hazards among adults in China. *Biomed Environ Sci.* 2010; 23(6): 437–444.
6. Yang G, Hu A. Tobacco Control and the Future of China. Beijing: The Economic Daily Press; 2011.
7. Yang L, Sung HY, Mao Z, Hu TW, Rao K. Economic costs attributable to smoking in China: update and an 8-year comparison, 2000–2008. *Tob Control.* 2011; 20(4): 266–272.
8. Yang G, Kong L, Zhao W, *et al.* Emergence of chronic non-communicable diseases in China. *Lancet.* 2008; 372(9650): 1697–1705.
9. Yang GH, Li Q, Wang CX, *et al.* Findings from 2010 Global Adult Tobacco Survey: implementation of MPOWER policy in China. *Biomed Environ Sci.* 2010; 23(6): 422–429.
10. Eriksen M, Mackey J, Ross H. The Tobacco Atlas. Atlanta, Georgia: American Cancer Society; 2012.

11. Full year analysis of national production of cigarettes 2010 (in Chinese). Available from: http://www.china-consulting.cn/article/html/2011/0527/101538.php (accessed 28 August, 2012).

12. Editorial. China advised to "put a brake" on tobacco industry. China Daily US Edition. 2011.

13. Editorial. Cost of Tobacco. China Daily US Edition. 2011.

14. China Tobacco. 2011 Report of the National Working Conference on tobacco. 2011. Available from: http://www.tobacco.gov.cn/html/48/4801/3662206_n.html (accessed 28 August, 2012).

15. www.people.com.cn. CNTC Daily Profits CNY 320 million Beijing2012. Available from: http://health.people.com.cn/GB/14740/22121/17311892.html (accessed 28 August, 2012).

16. www.china.com.cn. Total Government Revenue CNY10374 Billion, a 24.8% Increase Beijing 2012. Available from: http://finance.china.com.cn/news/gnjj/20120120/494751.shtml (accessed 28 August, 2012).

17. Li VC, Wang Q, Xia N, Tang S, Wang CC. Tobacco crop substitution: pilot effort in China. *Am J Public Health*. 2012; 102(9): 1660–1663.

18. Liu T, Xiong B. Tobacco Economy & Tobacco Control (in Chinese). Beijing: Economic Science Press; 2004.

19. National Bureau of Statistics of China. China Statistical Yearbook 2010. Beijing.

20. Yunnan Provincial Department of Finance. The report on the implementation of local budgets in 2010 and the local fiscal budget draft in 2011 in Yunnan Province. 2010.

21. Yunnan Provincial Government Information website of the Bureau of Statistics. 2010 report on economic development in Yunnan. 2010. Available from: www.stats.yn.gov.cn.

22. Lecours N, Almeida GE, Abdallah JM, Novotny TE. Environmental health impacts of tobacco farming: a review of the literature. *Tob Control*. 2012; 21(2): 191–196.

23. National Cancer Institute. Tobacco Companies' Public Relations Efforts: Corporate Sponsorship and Advertising. In: Davis R, Gilpin E, Loken B, Viswanath K, Wakefield M, (eds.). Tobacco Control Monograph 19: The Role of the Media in Promoting and Reducing Tobacco Use. Bethesda, MD: US Department of Health and Human Services; 2008, p. 179–209.

24. Hirschhorn N. Corporate social responsibility and the tobacco industry: hope or hype? *Tob Control*. 2004; 13(4): 447–453.

25. Xinhua News Agency. Ministry of Industry and Information Technology inaugurated. 2008. Available from: http://www.china.org.cn/government/news/2008-06/30/content_15906787.htm (accessed 22 May, 2013).

26. National Development and Research Council of China. State Tobacco Monopoly Administration (China National Tobacco Corporation). Available from: http://en.ndrc.gov.cn/mfod/t20050520_0881. htm (accessed 23 May, 2013).

27. TobaccoChina. 2013 New Year Address of Mr Jiang Chengkang, President of State Tobacco Monopoly Administration (in Chinese). Available from: http://en.ndrc.gov.cn/mfod/t20050520_0881.htm (accessed 21 May, 2013).

28. Lv J, Su M, Hong Z, *et al.* Implementation of the WHO Framework Convention on Tobacco Control in mainland China. *Tob Control*. 2011; 20(4): 309–314.

29. Wan X, Ma S, Hoek J, *et al*. Conflict of interest and FCTC implementation in China. *Tob Control*. 2012; 21(4): 412–415.

30. Chu A, Jiang N, Glantz SA. Transnational tobacco industry promotion of the cigarette gifting custom in China. *Tob Control*. 2011; 20(4): e3.

31. Hu TW, Mao Z, Shi J. Recent tobacco tax rate adjustment and its potential impact on tobacco control in China. *Tob Control*. 2010; 19(1): 80–82.

32. Warner KE. The economics of tobacco: myths and realities. *Tob Control*. 2000; 9(1): 78–89.

33. World Health Organization. WHO technical manual on tobacco tax administration. Geneva: WHO; 2010.

34. Pan Z. Socioeconomic predictors of smoking and smoking frequency in urban China: evidence of smoking as a social function. *Health Promot Int*. 2004; 19(3): 309–315.

35. Elton-Marshall T, Fong GT, Zanna MP, *et al*. Beliefs about the relative harm of "light" and "low tar" cigarettes: findings from the International Tobacco Control (ITC) China Survey. *Tob Control*. 2010; 19(Suppl 2i): 54–62.

36. World Health Organization. Gender, Women, and the Tobacco Epidemic. Geneva: WHO; 2010, p. 223–224.

37. Wasserman J, Manning WG, Newhouse JP, Winkler JD. The effects of excise taxes and regulations on cigarette smoking. *J Health Econ*. 1991; 10(1): 43–64.

38. cq.qq.com. Raising tobacco tax: experts have something to say (in Chinese). 2009. Available from: http://cq.qq.com/a/20090622/000412.htm (accessed 26 May, 2013).

39. Hu TW, Mao Z, Liu Y, de Beyer J, Ong M. Smoking, standard of living, and poverty in China. *Tob Control*. 2005; 14(4): 247–250.

40. Wang H. Tobacco control in China: the dilemma between economic development and health improvement. *Salud Publica Mex*. 2006; 48(Suppl 1): S140–S147.

41. Liu Y, Rao K, Hu TW, Sun Q, Mao Z. Cigarette smoking and poverty in China. *Soc Sci Med*. 2006; 63(11): 2784–2790.

42. Huang Y. The SARS epidemic and its aftermath in China: a political perspective. In: Knobler S, Mahmoud A, Lemon S, (eds.). Learning from SARS: Preparing for the Next Disease Outbreak: Workshop Summary, Institute of Medicine Forum on Microbial Threats. Washington DC: National Academies Press; 2004.

43. Champagne BM, Sebrie E, Schoj V. The role of organized civil society in tobacco control in Latin America and the Caribbean. *Salud Publica Mex*. 2010; 52(Suppl 2): S330–S339.

44. Hu TW, Mao Z, Jiang H, Tao M, Yurekli A. The role of government in tobacco leaf production in China: national and local interventions. *Int J Public Policy*. 2007; 2(3/4): 235–248.

Chapter 15

Tobacco Control in China: From Policy Research to Practice and the Way Forward

Teh-wei Hu and Xiulan Zhang

DISSEMINATION OF POLICY RESEARCH FINDINGS[a]

Since the 1990s, a group of international and Chinese economists have been actively advocating for increasing the retail price of cigarettes through raising the tax in China. With findings and support from international organizations, including the World Health Organization, World Bank, the US National Institutes of Health, Bloomberg Philanthropies, and the Gates Foundation, these economists published a series of studies on the economics of tobacco control in China. These studies have shown that raising the cigarette tax not only produces additional tax revenue, but it also saves lives and reduces medical costs by making smoking less financially viable for smokers (Hu, Mao, Shi, Chen, 2008; Hu, Mao, Shi, 2010; Gao, Zheng, Hu, 2011; Yang, Sung, Mao, 2011; Zheng, Gao, Hu, 2013; Levy *et al.*, 2014).

---

[a]A similar discussion was prepared by Teh-wei Hu who contributed to Chapter 7 entitled "Wrangling the cash cow: reforming tobacco taxation since Mao" (co-authored by Matthew Korhman, Gan Quan, and Teh-wei Hu), in *Poisonous Pandas and Pagodas: Critical Historical Perspective on Chinese Cigarette Manufacturing* (edited by M. Kohrman, Gan Quan, Liu Wennan, Robert Proctor), Stanford University Press, forthcoming.

Researchers recognized that persuading Chinese government policy-makers to adopt their policy recommendations would require extensive communication and exchanges. They presented their findings at numerous workshops in China between 2009 and 2014 at least once or twice a year, inviting key government officials from the Ministry of Health, Ministry of Finance, State Administration of Taxation, National Development and Reform Commission, State Council, the People's Congress, and the People's Political Consultation Conference. While these are important officials directly responsible for policy design and policy implementation in the Chinese government, they are not the decision makers in China because of the Chinese top-down decision-making process. The officials who attended the workshops could provide advice to the top leaders in the Chinese government and submit policy briefs to top government leaders. Once the leaders decided to increase tobacco taxes, these ministry officials could be ready to work with policy researchers to simulate the impact of various tobacco tax increase proposals on government revenue, the cigarette industry, and cigarette consumption.

Under China's top-down decision making process, the top government leaders had to be reached directly either through official channels, such as the People's Congress, the State Council, the Ministry of Health, or through private channels, such as the Chinese Association on Tobacco Control (CATC), the only nongovernmental organization on tobacco control in China. It turned out that the private personal connections with top government leaders were the most effective channel for the initiation of policy adaptation. Throughout the process, these researchers have been trying to leverage the World Health Organization's (WHO) Framework Convention on Tobacco Control (FCTC), the global health treaty that China rectified in 2005. A key provision of the FCTC is that member states should raise tax on cigarette and pass along to consumers, as one of the key tools for curbing cigarette smoking.

In addition to recognizing and working with the country's top-down approach to decision making, it was also important to utilize a bottom-up approach as suggested in the previous chapter (Hu, Lee, 2013). In close collaboration with CATC, researchers held numerous workshops each year and invited key newspapers and television reporters to learn from these research findings. Their news coverage would draw government leaders' attention as well as public opinion. For instance, a report (Hu, Mao, Shi, Chan, 2008) was released at a press conference in Beijing. This report suggested that raising the cigarette tax by 1 RMB ($0.15) per pack would lead 4 million smokers to quit smoking, saving one million premature deaths, and at the same time raising tax revenue for the Chinese government by 87 billion RMB, a win-win policy recommendation endorsed by *China Daily* (December 17, 2008). Those research findings became an international policy recommendation, often quoted by WHO and other Chinese tobacco control advocacy groups.

The 2009 tobacco tax adjustment helped the Chinese government raise tax revenue by transferring profits from the China National Tobacco Company, without raising the retail cigarette price. Thus, this tax adjustment had no effect on tobacco control. In 2010, economists published a study that showed the "effective tax" rate for a pack of cigarettes in China was well below the FCTC mandates. They estimated that the effective tax rate on a pack of cigarettes hovered somewhere between 40% and 43%, well below the WHO's 70% mandate (Hu, Mao, Shi, 2010). Seventy percent of cigarette tax on retail prices is considered as the best practice by WHO (WHO, 2010).

In late spring of 2014, tobacco-control economists organized a workshop in Beijing to celebrate the WHO World No Tobacco Day (May 31, 2014). They once again indicated at the workshop that cigarettes in China have a relatively low effective tax rate, between 43% to 49%, an estimate they based on Excise Tax and VAT data (Hu, Mao, Shi, 2010; Zheng, Gao, Hu, 2013; and Bai *et al.*, 2014). Within weeks, top economists from the China National Tobacco Corporation (CNTC) released a competing estimate to the news media and the State Council. The CNTC economists used a definition for calculating "effective rate" including not only Excise Tax and VAT, but also the corporate income tax, the supplemental education tax, and other important types of taxation that occurs in China tobacco industry. Using their calculations, the CNTC economists claimed that the average total tax on a retail pack of cigarettes was at 59.5%, considerably higher than the estimates by the tobacco-control economists (Yan, 2014). If government leaders were to agree that the relevant current average tax rate was nearly 60%, as CNTC economists claimed, then the leaders would see China as already having nearly met the WHO-recommended target tax rate of 70%. But if leaders agreed that the relevant current rate was considerably lower, as claimed by the tobacco-control economists, the Chinese government would likely resist on larger rate increases.

To resolve the disagreement over translational methodology between the two groups of economists, a workshop was organized by this research team. The chief economist and his colleagues at CNTC were invited to join economists from the tobacco control group for a dialogue on the tax rate issue. This was a unique workshop in that the WHO has a policy of not meeting with tobacco industry officials. In this case, the China CDC tobacco control officials served as workshop arrangers to discuss the methodology for calculating the tobacco tax rate. At an October 2014 workshop in Beijing, representatives from the CNTC, the Ministry of Finance, and the State Administration of Taxation agreed to adopt the WHO-endorsed method used by the tobacco-prevention economists. Shortly after the workshop concluded, the Chinese President's Central Administrative Office requested the tobacco-control economists to provide a policy brief.

POLICY BRIEF SUBMITTED TO THE PRESIDENT'S OFFICE

The policy brief was prepared by a group of economists who attended the workshop.[b] The purposes of the policy brief submitted to President Xi's Central Administrative Office were to clarify the status of tobacco excise tax levels in China and assess the opportunity to increase the tobacco tax, as well as offer suggestions on tobacco taxation policy in China. The policy brief consists of five sections: (1) Chinese excise tax level using the WHO calculating standard, (2) huge room for increasing tobacco excise in China, (3) impact of raising tobacco tax on tobacco consumption, fiscal revenue, population health, tobacco industry, tax burden on low-income smoker and potential brand switch, (4) international experiences, and (5) policy recommendations. A brief summary of these sections follows:

1. Chinese Tobacco Excise Tax Level Using the WHO Calculating Standard

According to the WHO Technical Manual on Tobacco Taxes Administration, tobacco taxation refers to the taxes imposed on all tobacco products such as cigarettes, cigars, and other tobacco products during the process of tobacco

---

[b]They are Hu Teh-wei, Professor Emeritus of University of California, Berkeley, and Director of the Center for International Tobacco Control Policy, the Public Health Institute; Zhang Xiulan, Professor of School of Social Development and Public Policy, Beijing Normal University; Zheng Rong, Professor of University of International Business and Economics; Shi Jian, Director of Fiscal Scientific Research Institute, State Administration of Taxation (People's Republic of China); Liang Ji, Researcher of Research Institute for Fiscal Science (RIFS), Ministry of Finance (People's Republic of China); Yang Gonghuan, Professor of Institute of Basic Medical, Chinese Academy of Medical Sciences; and Jiang Yuan, Deputy Director of China Center for Disease Control and Prevention.

production and sales. In most countries, these taxes are the value-added and excise tax, and they also include customs duties on tobacco imports. Raising the tobacco excise tax is the major leverage for increasing the price of tobacco products, as the others do not contribute directly to fluctuations in the retail price of these products.

In China, tobacco product taxation includes taxes on tobacco leaf, value-added and excise taxes. It also includes the value-added urban construction and maintenance taxes, and an additional educational tax. Moreover, a general enterprise income tax is imposed on all tobacco-related commercial enterprises, including tobacco producing and selling enterprises. Income tax should not be counted in calculating the tobacco tax, since it was corporate revenue after the product was sold and it does not affect the retail price of cigarettes. The amount of profit is actually influenced by the price on the market. Similarly, because tobacco enterprises are state-owned in China, the portion of their profit that is turned in to the government should not be counted either. The method for calculating the tobacco tax in China should abide by the WHO definition. Using the WHO calculating standard, the actual tobacco tax in China is between 40%–49%.

Economists at the China National Tobacco Company (CNTC) reported that total tobacco tax in China is 59.5%. This percentage includes all taxes submitted to the government in 2013. Obviously, CNTC's calculation of its tobacco taxation is very different from the calculation using the WHO definition, which refers specifically to a tobacco consumption tax. In the Tobacco Tax Conference held by the Tobacco Control Office of the Chinese Center for Disease Control and Prevention (CDC) on October 22, 2014, all the experts, including those from China's tobacco enterprises, agreed to use the WHO definition to calculate the tobacco tax.

2. Huge Room for Increasing Tobacco Excise Tax in China

On October 15, 2014, Guidelines for Implementation of Article 6 of the FCTC were approved by the sixth session of the Conference of Parties. Using the accumulated empirical evidence on tobacco tax practices that have successfully reduced cigarette consumption in some ratified counties, the WHO recommends that the tobacco excise tax should represent at least 70% of the retail price of tobacco products. Given the effective tobacco tax rate is close to 46%, a huge amount of room exists for increasing the tobacco excise tax in China.

Table 1:   Retail Prices of Tobacco and Other Foods in China

Year	Food	Tea & Drinks	Tobacco	Alcohol
2000	100	100	100	100
2001	100	99.1	99.6	99.9
2002	99.4	98.1	99.5	100
2003	102.8	97.3	99.3	100.1
2004	113	97.1	100	102.3
2005	116.2	97.2	100.4	102.9
2006	119.3	98.2	100.6	104.3
2007	133.9	99.6	101.5	107.8
2008	153.2	103.4	102	115.9
2009	154.6	105.3	102.4	119.7
2010	166.3	106.9	102.9	124.1
2011	186.1	111.1	103.3	132.6
2012	195.1	115.5	103.9	140.9

Source: China National Bureau of Statistics, *China National Statistical Yearbook, 2000–2013*. Beijing, China.

As shown in Table 1 and Figure 1, cigarette prices in China did not increase much during the past decade. According to the China National Statistics Yearbook, from 2000 to 2012, the price index of cigarettes rose by just 4 percent (year 2000 = 100, 2012 = 103.9). In contrast, food prices doubled (2000 = 100, 2012 = 195.1), the alcohol price index increased 40 percent (2000 = 100, 2012 = 140.9), and the price of tea and soft drinks went up 15 percent (2000 = 100, 2012 = 115.5). Therefore, the rate of increase of cigarette prices is way behind that of many other food consumption products.

Furthermore, China made rapid economic growth between 2000 and 2012, with an annual rate of GDP growth of more than 9%. If one includes per capita income together with the price increase in cigarettes, the affordability index of cigarette consumption in China between 2000 and 2012 actually increased from 1.00 in 2000 to 1.69, an almost 70% increase in purchasing power, as shown in Table 2 and Figure 2. Therefore, ample room remains for the Chinese government to further increase the tax on cigarettes.

3. Impact of Raising the Tobacco Tax on Tobacco Consumption, Fiscal Revenue, Population Health, Tobacco Industry, and Low-income Smokers.

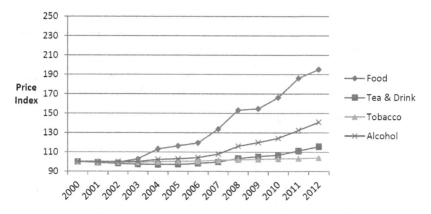

Fig 1: Retail Prices of Tobacco and Other Foods in China (year 2000 = 100)

Source: China National Tobacco Company, *China Tobacco Statistics Yearbook*, 2000–2013. Beijing, China.
China National Bureau of Statistics, *China National Statistical Yearbook*, 2000–2013. Beijing, China.

To make informative policy decisions, it's important to address the potential impacts of raising the tobacco tax on various aspects of the Chinese economy.

(1) Tobacco Consumption, Fiscal Revenue, and Population Health.
A basic principle in economics is that when price goes up, consumption goes down. The relationship between these two is called price-related elasticity of demand, which measures the response of demand to a price change. Tax is a part of price. Economic analyses have shown that the price elasticity of the demand for cigarettes ranges from −0.15 to −0.50. At a cigarette consumption elasticity of −0.15 to −0.50, a 1 Yuan increase in a specific duty (or specific tariff) will reduce consumption by 3.1 billion packs, 4 million smokers will quit smoking, and 1 million lives will be saved. Though the quantity of tobacco consumption will decrease with the tax increase, government revenues will increase by 85.4 billion Yuan because the rate of tax increase is greater than the rate of consumption decrease (Hu, Mao, Shi, Chen, 2008).
(2) Tobacco Industry and Farming
Tobacco enterprises and tobacco farmers may worry that raising the tobacco tax will negatively impact their employment and income in a

Table 2: The Affordability Index of Cigarette Consumption (2000–2012)

Year	Nominal Cigarette Price (Yuan/pack)	Consumer Price Index (1990 = 100)	Actual Cigarette Price (Yuan/pack)	Per-capita Disposal Income (Yuan)	Affordability Index
2000	2.585	200.5	1.289	7732	1.988
2001	2.793	201.9	1.383	8467	2.015
2002	3.086	200.3	1.541	9271	1.997
2003	3.42	202.7	1.687	10460	2.033
2004	3.899	210.6	1.851	12277	2.093
2005	4.522	214.4	2.109	14128	2.076
2006	4.628	217.6	2.127	13475	2.328
2007	5.406	228.1	2.371	16279	2.34
2008	5.427	241.5	2.247	19122	2.342
2009	5	239.8	2.085	20448	2.718
2010	5.4	247.7	2.18	23876	2.938
2011	5.422	269.7	2.01	24207	2.967
2012	5.427	291.7	1.86	27437	3.36

Source: China National Tobacco Company, *China Tobacco Statistics Yearbook, 2000–2013*. Beijing, China.
China National Bureau of Statistics, *China National Statistical Yearbook, 2000–2013*. Beijing, China.

significant way. As noted above, based on the relationship between the cost and output of the cigarette industry, a 1 Yuan increase in the tobacco tax will reduce consumption by 3.1 billion packs. In turn, this increase will lead to a reduction of 1,656 employees in the tobacco industry, just 2% to 3% of the 60,000 who retire or are laid off each year. Similarly, the decreased consumption of 3.1 billion packs will lead to a decline of 26,000 tons of tobacco leaf production, only 1% of the national yearly yield of tobacco (2.43 million tons in 2005). Meanwhile, tobacco leaf is not the most economically beneficial crop; other crops such as fruit trees and vegetable oils will bring farmers more income. Therefore, the short-run negative influence of raising the tobacco tax will be negligible (Hu, Mao, Shi, Chen, 2008).

(3) Economic Burden on Low-income Smokers

People may worry that raising the tobacco tax will further aggravate the economic burden of low-income smokers, which already is unfair.

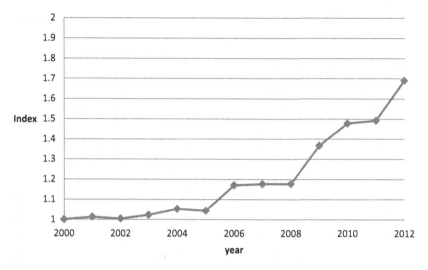

Fig 2: The Affordability Index of Cigarette Consumption (2000–2012)

The government has increased the income subsidy for low-income families in recent years. Compared with the high-income group, low-income families are more sensitive to a tobacco price increase. Thus, when the tobacco tax rises, low-income individuals will likely cease smoking or buy fewer cigarettes, so more money will be available for family household consumption. Moreover, low-income individuals will benefit more from the social welfare expenditures collected from the tobacco tax.

(4) Potential Brand-switch

In China, the price of different cigarettes varies largely, from 2 Yuan to over 100 Yuan per pack. Some officials believe that smokers will turn to a lower-priced product when the tobacco tax goes up, resulting in minimal impact on smoking behavior. Thus, these people consider that raising the tax would not have an effect on reducing cigarette consumption. However, according to a panel data analysis that followed 5,000 people in six cities from 2006 to 2009, only about 7% to 8% of smokers will turn to lower-priced tobacco products when the price of cigarettes rises (Li, White, Hu, Jiang, Fong, 2015).

In summary, raising the tobacco tax will reduce tobacco consumption, increase fiscal revenue, promote population health, and cut down on health expenditures. The negative impacts on the tobacco industry and farmers are minimal.

4. International Experiences

The WHO Technical Manual on Tobacco Tax Administration (WHO, 2010) shows that of 186 countries, 60 countries impose only an ad valorem tax on tobacco products, 55 countries have adopted a specific excise tax, and 84 countries have both specific and ad valorem taxes. Currently, China imposes both a specific tax and an ad valorem tax. Based on relevant theories and practical experiences, a specific excise tax is better than an ad valorem tax with respect to preventing tobacco manufacturers from evading tax action by transferring pricing strategies. The specific tax is minimally influenced by price fluctuation and variations. Thus, compared with an ad valorem tax, the specific tax will play a more significant role in increasing the price of tobacco products.

In terms of the efficiency of administering the taxation, a single rate tax is easier to administer and more transparent for the public than multi-layer taxation. A single rate tax can prevent consumers from substituting brands and will help improve collection of tax revenue. If there are two specific excise tax rates for two different tobacco products, tobacco producers may be induced to produce to their lower tax rate brand strategy.

Regarding the management of tobacco tax administration, the WHO Technical Manual on Tobacco Tax Administration shows that more than 20 countries have allocated part or all of their tobacco tax revenue to public health service, health insurance, or tobacco control programs. This strategy is the win-win practice for tobacco control programs. In the United States, California has earmarked part of its tobacco tax revenue into a special fund for tobacco control programs; these programs have significantly reduced the numbers of smokers in California. The following are some similar examples from around the world in the last five years.

The United States. The tobacco tax in the United States consists of a local tax (state tax) and a federal tax; both taxes are levied at the retail level. The local tax, which is levied by state governments, has different rates in different states,. The federal tax has a uniform rate, which is levied as a specific excise tax. Before 2009, the federal tax was 39 cents per pack. It rose to $1.01 per pack in 2009, an increase of 62 cents. The sales volume in 2009 was 8.3% lower than in 2008, but the tax revenue increased by $1,276 million from 2008. The government used that revenue to provide health insurance for 8 million adolescents.

France. France's Finance Ministry increased the tobacco tax by 30 cents per pack in October 2011, raising the price of cigarettes by 6%. The sales volume had dropped 4.3% from October 2010 to June 2012. In October 2012, the National Parliament further raised the tobacco tax by 4.5% to subsidize the country's social security fund in 2013.

Hong Kong and Macao. In recent years, Hong Kong and Macao have dramatically increased their tobacco tax. Hong Kong increased the tax by 8 HK dollars per pack in 2009 and further to 10 HK dollars per pack in 2011, raising the cost from 39 HK dollars per pack to 49 HK dollars per pack. That makes the tobacco tax 68% of the tobacco retail price. Most of the increased revenues are used for health services, health service research, and tobacco control. The Macao government increased the tobacco tax from 4 Macao dollars per pack in 2009 to 10 Macao dollars in 2011. As a result, the tobacco tax represents 55% of the retail price of a pack of cigarettes in Macao.

Taiwan. Taiwan has begun to use the tobacco tax as an effective tool for tobacco control and to subsidize health care. In 2006, Taiwan increased its tobacco tax by 10 NTD per pack, and in 2009 by another 10 NTD per pack. The additional revenue is used for health welfare (70%) and for cancer treatment, tobacco control, and smoking cessation (30%). In 2011, the tobacco tax in Taiwan accounted for 53% of the retail price.

Since China signed the FCTC in 2005, many countries, including Turkey, Japan, Egypt, India, Brazil, Singapore, Thailand, Philippines, and Australia have increased their tobacco tax. These countries generally have had successful experiences, which can be very valuable examples for China. The lessons from the experiences of other countries are summarized as follows:

- Raising the tobacco tax is the most effective policy tool for tobacco control. It can successfully reduce tobacco consumption and encourage smoking cessation, further improving the quality of public health.
- As the tobacco tax constitutes an increased proportion of the retail price of cigarettes, the specific excise tax on tobacco becomes more efficient and reliable than the ad valorem tax for raising government revenue.
- Increasing the tobacco tax by a one-time larger amount is more efficient than multiple increases of smaller amounts. A single large increase also significantly reduces the administrative cost.

- In China, the tobacco tax should reach at least the level of the international level, namely, 70%, according to the WHO recommendation.
- A portion of the tobacco tax revenue should be used for health services and tobacco control.

5. Policy Recommendations

Scientific evidence shows that smoking is harmful to health and increases tremendously the costs of health care. Raising the tobacco tax is the most effective tobacco control policy tool and will improve fiscal revenue. In China, although the smoking prevalence rate is going down gradually, the number of smokers will not decrease notably due to the continuous increase in population. China's tobacco enterprises will be influenced very little by tobacco control activities in the near future. Currently, the tobacco tax in China is quite low, suggesting a vast amount of room exists for increasing the tobacco tax.

Based on the above discussion, the authors offer the following recommendations:

(1) Increase the specific tax on tobacco products

The current specific tax of 0.06 Yuan per pack at the producer price level is too low to have any substantive influence on tobacco control and fiscal revenue in China. Reform of the excise tax system is now on the Chinese government's policy agenda, The Chinese government should take the opportunity to increase the tobacco specific tax by at least 1 Yuan per pack and levy it at the retail level. This measure will be the most effective policy tool for tobacco control in China. Since does not have a retail sales tax collection system to reduce administrative cost, the tax could be levied at the wholesale level. The wholesalers would collect the tax for the government. In the long run, the specific excise tax should be increased to 4 Yuan per pack so that the tobacco tax will reach 70%, the level recommended by the WHO.

(2) Unify the rate of the ad valorem tax

To prevent the industry from avoiding a higher tax by selling lower-priced brands, the ad valorem tax on cigarettes should be set at a uniform rate for all categories of cigarettes, the current rate for category A cigarettes, which is 56%, category B cigarettes is levied at 36% of the producer price. A single rate of 56% would save much of the administrative cost of tax collection.

(3) Earmark additional tax revenue

The government should earmark the added tax revenue to subsidize tobacco farmers to develop other cash crops and improve their ability to substitute other crops for tobacco. The additional revenue also can be used to provide health insurance for the low-income population and support tobacco control programs. By combining the tax policy with nonprice tobacco control mechanisms (e.g., legislation mandating smoke-free public areas and providing larger warning labels), tobacco control efforts in China will have a much better outcome.

POLICY ADOPTION

On May 8, 2015, the Chinese Ministry of Finance announced the following changes effective May 11, 2015: (1) an increase in the ad valorem tax rate on cigarettes at the wholesale price level from 5% to 11%, and (2) an additional specific excise tax of 0.10 RMB ($0.016) per pack of cigarettes at the wholesale price level. In the meantime, the China State Tobacco Monopoly Administration (STMA) announced that the wholesale prices of all cigarettes would be increased by 6%; the local STMAs will decide how much to increase the retail price of cigarettes. Table 3 compares China's tobacco excise tax rates before and after May 10, 2015. These combined excise tax rate changes shifted to the retail price will increase the average retail price of cigarettes by close to 1 RMB ($0.16) per pack, which will raise the total share of taxes from 49% to 54% of the average retail price. It is estimated that as a result of the

Table 3:   Comparison of Chinese Tobacco Tax Structure before and after May 10, 2015

	Before May 10, 2015	After May 10, 2015
At Producer price level		
Specific excise tax (per pack)	0.06 RMB	0.06 RMB
Ad valorem tax		
>= 7 RMB	56%	56%
<7 RMB	36%	36%
At Wholesale price level		
Specific excise tax (per pack)	0	0.10 RMB
Ad valorem tax	5%	11%

tax increases, the Chinese government will raise close to an additional 100 billion RMB, depending on the estimated price elasticities of the demand for cigarettes, which range between −0.15 and −0.40. The China National Tobacco Company predicted their sales could be reduced between 2 billion and 2.25 billion packs (Xu, 2015). From the public health point of view, depending on the magnitude of the price elasticities, the tax increase would lead 2 million smokers to quit smoking (and many youth would not initiate smoking). Therefore, the tax increase is welcome news for tobacco control communities.

Under the 2009 Chinese tobacco tax adjustment, the tax revenue for the government came from tobacco companies rather than consumers. The tax adjustment in 2009 specifically forbade shifting the tax increase to the cigarette retail price (Hu, Mao, Shi, 2010). This time, the Chinese government declared its commitment, 10 years after China's ratification of the World Health Organization (WHO) Framework Convention on Tobacco Central, to comply with Article 6 of the FCTC, which calls for raising the tobacco tax and shifting the tax increase to the retail price level.

The recent tax adjustment has moved the increase from the tax base at the producer price level to the wholesale price level, making it easier to pass along the tax increase to the retail price level. Furthermore, the Chinese government has adopted a specific excise tax at the wholesale price level, instead of at the producer price level, although the amount of the increase is quite minimal. The WHO Tobacco Tax Administration Manual has suggested that the use of a specific excise tax is more efficient for tax collection and more effective for tobacco control (WHO, 2010).

Finally, the recent tax adjustment will change the pricing structure of the five classes of cigarette products. Raising the ad valorem tax for all classes will reduce the market share of the lowest brand (class V) and eventually eliminate sales of the lowest priced brand of cigarettes. Raising the price across all brands will increase the overall price of cigarettes by 7.3%, about additional 1 RMB per pack.

THE WAY FORWARD

Using a tobacco tax as an instrument for tobacco control is a significant step for the Chinese government. However, the increase in the resulting tax rate as a percentage of the retail price, from 49% to 56%, is still relatively low compared to the WHO-recommended benchmark, which is about 70% of the retail price. Therefore, ample room remains for the Chinese government to further increase the tax on cigarettes.

While the May 11, 2015, tax increase in China was welcome news, the government adopted only the first part of the recommendations suggested in the policy brief submitted to President Xi's office, increasing the tax by only 0.05 Yuan per pack (not the 1 Yuan per pack increase suggested in the policy brief) at the wholesale price level. The government did raise the ad valorem tax at the wholesale price level to 11%, but did not unify the tax rate for category A and category B cigarettes. Finally, the government did not earmark part of the additional tax revenue for health care reform or for tobacco control.

Since the China National Tobacco Company has a major political and economic role within the Chinese government, increasing the tobacco tax rate requires multiple government agencies to negotiate, give, and take for the interest of each of the stakeholders. Achieving the goal of tobacco tax increase up to 70% of the retail price may take longer than tobacco control advocates would wish. Some recommendations suggested in the policy brief submitted to President Xi's office still need to be adopted.

As shown in Table 3, China has a very complicated tobacco tax structure. The Ministry of Finance is still undergoing overall excise tax reform. Following the WHO Tobacco Tax Administration guideline (WHO, 2010), the next round of tobacco tax reform in China hopefully will involve simplifying its tobacco tax structure by (1) raising the specific excise tax at the wholesale price level from 0.05 RMB to 1.00 RMB per pack, and (2) converting the tiered ad valorem tax rates into a uniform tax rate, such as raising the tax rate from 36% to 56% for all classes of cigarette products. With these suggested additional tax increase, China would be reaching the WHO recommended benchmark, close to 70% of the retail price.

China has been making good progress on health care insurance reform. However, additional revenue is needed to sustain the country's health care services delivery. As is the case with many other countries, such as the Philippines, Thailand, the United States, Australia, and others, China could justify allocating a portion of these additional tobacco tax revenues for healthcare services, tobacco control mechanisms, and environmental improvement so that lower-income people including smokers would benefit.

Finally, it will be very important to conduct empirical evaluations of the impact of this recent tobacco tax increase on changes in cigarette consumption, smoking behavior, retail cigarette prices, market structure of brand shares, and changes in government revenues. Findings of these analyses would be useful for the next round of tobacco tax policy adjustment.

Funding: This study is funded by the U.S. National Institute of Health, Fogarty International Center Grant (R01-TW009295), and the Bill and Melinda Gates Foundation support to the Beijing Normal University.

REFERENCES

1. Bai, J. "Production cost of Chinese Tobacco Industry and analysis of Its Pricing and Mechanism." Presentation at a Conference on Economics of Tobacco Control, May 29, 2014. A report prepared by Bai *et al.* from the Research Institute of Public Finance. Source, Ministry of Finance, China.
2. China National Bureau of Statistics, *China National Statistical Year Book*, 2000–2013. Beijing, China.
3. China National Tobacco Company, *China Tobacco Statistics Year Book* (2000–2013). Beijing, China.
4. Gao S, Zheng R, Hu TW. Can increases in the cigarette tax rate be linked to cigarette retail prices? Solving mysteries related to the cigarette pricing mechanism in China. Tobacco Control 2011; DOI: 10.1136/tobaccocontrol-2011-050027.
5. Hu T-w, Mao Z, Shih J., Chen WD. Tobacco Taxation and Its Potential Impact in China. Paris: International Union against Tuberculosis and Lung disease; Oct 2008.
6. Hu T-w, Mao Z, Shi J. Recent Tobacco Tax Rate Adjustment and Its Potential Impact on Tobacco Control in China. Tobacco Control 2010; 19(1): 80–82.
7. Levy D, Rodriguez-Buno RL, Hu TW, Moran AE. The potential effects of tobacco control in China: Projections from the China SimSmoke simulation model. BMJ. 2014 Feb 18; 348: g1134.
8. World Health Organization, WHO Technical Manual on Tobacco Tax Administration. Geneva, Switzerland, 2010.
9. Xu Y.B., Another Round of Tobacco Tax Reform, Tobacco Industry Will Face Major Revolution (in Chinese) http://www.yancaotx.com/article-105-1.html accessed on 6/16/2015.
10. Yan, D. A debate on using Tax as a means for Tobacco Control between Tobacco Industry and Tobacco Control Advocacy Group: A Full of Hope but Shivering in Reality," *South China Weekend* (in Chinese), July 4, 2014.
11. Yang L, Sung HY, Mao Z, Hu TW, Rao K. Economic costs attributable to smoking in China; an update and an 8-year comparison, 2000–2008. Tobacco Control 2011; 20(4): 266–272.
12. Zheng R, Gao S, Hu T. "Tobacco Tax and Tobacco Control — Global Experiences from WHO Tobacco Tax Technical Management Handbook and Challenges for China Tobacco Control," *Increase Tobacco Consumption Tax Policy Research* (edited by Shi J and Hu T). China Taxation Press (in Chinese), Beijing, 2013, pp. 183–204.

Index

Printed in the United States
By Bookmasters